T0094176

Surgery: Complications, Risks and Consequences

Series Editor
Brendon J. Coventry

For further volumes:
http://www.springer.com/series/11761

Brendon J. Coventry

Editor

Peripheral, Head and Neck Surgery

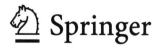 Springer

Editor
Brendon J. Coventry, BMBS, PhD, FRACS,
FACS, FRSM
Discipline of Surgery
Royal Adelaide Hospital
University of Adelaide
Adelaide, SA
Australia

ISBN 978-1-4471-5414-3   ISBN 978-1-4471-5415-0   (eBook)
DOI 10.1007/978-1-4471-5415-0
Springer London Heidelberg New York Dordrecht

Library of Congress Control Number: 2013956935

This book is dedicated to my wonderful wife Christine and children Charles, Cameron, Alexander and Eloise who make me so proud, having supported me through this mammoth project; my patients, past, present and future; my numerous mentors, teachers, colleagues, friends and students, who know who they are; my parents Beryl and Lawrence; and my parents-in-law Barbara and George, all of whom have taught me and encouraged me to achieve

"Without love and understanding we have but nothing"

Brendon J. Coventry

Foreword I

This comprehensive treatise is remarkable for its breadth and scope and its authorship by global experts. Indeed, knowledge of its content is essential if we are to achieve optimal and safe outcomes for our patients. The content embodies the details of our surgical discipline and how to incorporate facts and evidence into our surgical judgment as well as recommendations to our patients.

While acknowledging that the technical aspects of surgery are its distinguishing framework of our profession, the art and judgment of surgery requires an in depth knowledge of biology, anatomy, pathophysiology, clinical science, surgical outcomes and complications that distinguishes the theme of this book. This knowledge is essential to assure us that we are we doing the right operation, at the right time, and in the right patient. In turn, that knowledge is essential to take into account how surgical treatment interfaces with the correct sequence and combination with other treatment modalities. It is also essential to assess the extent of scientific evidence from clinical trials and surgical expertise that is the underpinning of our final treatment recommendation to our patient.

Each time I sit across from a patient to make a recommendation for a surgical treatment, I am basing my recommendation on a "benefit/risk ratio" that integrates scientific evidence, and my intuition gained through experience. That is, do the potential benefits outweigh the potential risks and complications as applied to an individual patient setting? The elements of that benefit/ risk ratio that are taken into account include: the natural history of the disease, the stage/extent of disease, scientific and empirical evidence of treatment outcomes, quality of life issues (as perceived by the patient), co-morbidity that might influence surgical outcome, risks and complications inherent to the operation (errors of commission) and the risk(s) of not proceeding with an operation (errors of omission).

Thus, if we truly want to improve our surgical outcomes, then we must understand and be able to either avoid, or execute sound management of, any complications that occur (regardless of whether they are due to co-morbidity or iatrogenic causes), to get our patent safely through the operation and its post-operative course. These subjects are nicely incorporated into the content of this book.

I highly recommend this book as a practical yet comprehensive treatise for the practicing surgeon and the surgical trainee. It is well organized, written with great clarity and nicely referenced when circumstances require further information.

Charles M. Balch, MD, FACS
Professor of Surgery
University of Texas, Southwestern Medical Center,
Dallas, TX, USA
Formerly, Professor of Surgery, Johns Hopkins Hospital,
Baltimore, MD, USA
Formerly, Executive Vice President and CEO,
American Society of Clinical Oncology (ASCO)
Past-President, Society of Surgical Oncology (USA)

Foreword II

Throughout my clinical academic career I have aspired to improve the quality and safety of my surgical and clinical practice. It is very clear, while reading this impressive collection and synthesis of high-impact clinical evidence and international expert consensus, that in this new textbook, Brendon Coventry has the ambition to innovate and advance the quality and safety of surgical discipline.

In these modern times, where we find an abundance of information that is available through the internet, and of often doubtful authenticity, it is vital that we retain a professional responsibility for the collection, analysis and dissemination of evidenced-based and accurate knowledge and guidance to benefit both clinicians and our patients.

This practical and broad-scoped compendium, which contains over 250 procedures and their related complications and associated risks, will undoubtedly become a benchmark to raise the safety and quality of surgical practice for all that read it. It also manages to succeed in providing a portal for all surgeons, at any stage of their careers, to reflect on the authors' own combined experiences and the collective insights of a strong and influential network of peers.

This text emphasizes the need to understand and appreciate our patients and the intimate relationship that their physiology, co-morbidities and underlying diagnosis can have upon their unique surgical risk with special regard to complications and adverse events.

I recognize that universally across clinical practice and our profession, the evidence base and guidance to justify our decision-making is growing, but there is also a widening gap between what we know and what we do. The variation that we see in the quality of practice throughout the world should not be tolerated.

This text makes an assertive contribution to promote quality by outlining the prerequisite foundational knowledge of surgery, science and anatomy and their complex interactions with clinical outcome that is needed for all in the field of surgery.

I thoroughly recommend this expertly constructed collection. Its breadth and quality is a testament to its authors and editor.

Professor the Lord Ara Darzi, PC, KBE, FRCS, FRS
Paul Hamlyn Chair of Surgery
Imperial College London, London, UK
Formerly Undersecretary of State for Health,
Her Majesty's Government, UK

Conditions of Use and Disclaimer

Information is provided *for improved medical education and potential improvement in clinical practice only*. The information is based on composite material from research studies and professional personal opinion and does not guarantee accuracy for any specific clinical situation or procedure. There is also *no express or implied guarantee to accuracy or that surgical complications will be prevented, minimized, or reduced* in any way. The advice is *intended for use by individuals with suitable professional qualifications* and education in medical practice and the ability to apply the knowledge in a suitable manner for a specific condition or disease, and in an appropriate clinical context. The data is complex by nature and open to some interpretation. The purpose is to assist medical practitioners to improve awareness of possible complications, risks or consequences associated with surgical procedures for the benefit of those practitioners in the improved care of their patients. The application of the information contained herein for a specific patient or problem must be performed with care to ensure that the situation and advice is appropriate and correct for that patient and situation. The material is expressly *not for medicolegal purposes*.

The information contained in *Surgery: Complications, Risks and Consequences* is provided for the purpose of improving consent processes in healthcare and in no way guarantees prevention, early detection, risk reduction, economic benefit or improved practice of surgical treatment of any disease or condition.

The information provided in *Surgery: Complications, Risks and Consequences* is of a general nature and is not a substitute for independent medical advice or research in the management of particular diseases or patient situations by health care professionals. It should not be taken as replacing or overriding medical advice.

The Publisher or *Copyright* holder does not accept any liability for any injury, loss, delay or damage incurred arising from use, misuse, interpretation, omissions or reliance on the information provided in *Surgery: Complications, Risks and Consequences* directly or indirectly.

Currency and Accuracy of Information

The user should always check that any information acted upon is up-to-date and accurate. Information is provided in good faith and is **subject to change and alteration without notice**. Every effort is made with *Surgery: Complications, Risks and Consequences* to provide current information, but no warranty, guarantee or legal responsibility is given that information provided or referred to has not changed without the knowledge of the publisher, editor or authors. Always check the quality of information provided or referred to for accuracy for the situation where it is intended to be used, or applied. We do, however, attempt to provide useful and valid information. Because of the broad nature of the information provided incompleteness or omissions of specific or general complications may have occured and users must take this into account when using the text. No responsibility is taken for delayed, missed or inaccurate diagnosis of any illness, disease or health state at any time.

External Web Site Links or References

The decisions about the accuracy, currency, reliability and correctness of information made by individuals using the *Surgery: Complications, Risks and Consequences* information or from external Internet links remain the individuals own concern and responsibility. Such external links or reference materials or other information should not be taken as an endorsement, agreement or recommendation of any third party products, services, material, information, views or content offered by these sites or publications. Users should check the sources and validity of information obtained for themselves prior to use.

Privacy and Confidentiality

We maintain confidentiality and privacy of personal information but do not guarantee any confidentiality or privacy.

Errors or Suggested Changes

If you or any colleagues note any errors or wish to suggest changes please notify us directly as they would be gratefully received.

How to Use This Book

This book provides a resource for better understanding of surgical procedures and potential complications in general terms. The application of this material will depend on the individual patient and clinical context. It is not intended to be absolutely comprehensive for all situations or for all patients, but act as a 'guide' for understanding and prediction of complications, to assist in risk management and improvement of patient outcomes.

The design of the book is aimed at:

- Reducing Risk and better Managing Risks associated with surgery
- Providing information about 'general complications' associated with surgery
- Providing information about 'specific complications' associated with surgery
- Providing comprehensive information in one location, to assist surgeons in their explanation to the patient during the consent process

For each specific surgical procedure the text provides:

- Description and some background of the surgical procedure
- Anatomical points and possible variations
- Estimated Frequencies
- Perspective
- Major Complications

From this, a better understanding of the risks, complications and consequences associated with surgical procedures can hopefully be gained by the clinician for explanation of relevant and appropriate aspects to the patient.

The *Estimated frequency lists are not mean't to be totally comprehensive* or to contain all of the information that needs to be explained in obtaining informed consent from the patient for a surgical procedure. Indeed, *most of the information is for the surgeon* or reader only, *not designed for the patient*, however, parts should be selected by the surgeon at their discretion for appropriate explanation to the individual patient in the consent process.

Many patients would not understand or would be confused by the number of potential complications that may be associated with a specific surgical procedure, so ***some degree of selective discussion of the risks, complications and consequences would be necessary and advisable***, as would usually occur in clinical practice. This judgement should necessarily be left to the surgeon, surgeon-in-training or other practitioner.

Preface

Over the last decade or so we have witnessed a rapid change in the consumer demand for information by patients preparing for a surgical procedure. This is fuelled by multiple factors including the 'internet revolution', altered public consumer attitudes, professional patient advocacy, freedom of information laws, insurance issues, risk management, and medicolegal claims made through the legal system throughout the western world, so that the need has arisen for a higher, fairer and clearer standard of *'informed consent'*.

One of the my main difficulties encountered as a young intern, and later as a surgical resident, registrar and consultant surgeon, was obtaining information for use for the pre-operative consenting of patients, and for managing patients on the ward after surgical operations. I watched others struggle with the same problem too. The literature contained many useful facts and clinical studies, but it was unwieldy and very time-consuming to access, and the information that was obtained seemed specific to well-defined studies of highly specific groups of patients. These patient studies, while useful, often did not address my particular patient under treatment in the clinic, operating theatre or ward. Often the studies came from centres with vast experience of a particular condition treated with one type of surgical procedure, constituting a series or trial.

What I wanted to know was:

- The **main complications** associated with a surgical procedure;
- **Information that could be provided** during the consent process, and
- How to **reduce the relative risks** of a complication, where possible

This information was difficult to find in one place!

As a young surgeon, on a very long flight from Adelaide to London, with much time to think and fuelled by some very pleasant champagne, I started making some notes about how I might tackle this problem. My first draft was idle scribble, as I listed the ways surgical complications could be classified. After finding over 10 different classification systems for listing complications, the task became much larger and more complex. I then realized why someone had not taken on this job before!

After a brief in-flight sleep and another glass, the task became far less daunting and suddenly much clearer – the champagne was very good, and there was little else to do in any case!

It was then that I decided to speak with as many of my respected colleagues as I could from around the globe, to get their opinions and advice. The perspectives that emerged were remarkable, as many of them had faced the same dilemmas in their own practices and hospitals, also without a satisfactory solution.

What developed was a composite documentation of information (i) from the published literature and (ii) from the opinions of many experienced surgical practitioners in the field – to provide a text to supply information on **Complications, Risks and Consequences of Surgery** for surgical and other clinical practitioners to use at the bedside and in the clinic.

This work represents the culmination of more than 10 years work with the support and help of colleagues from around the world, for the benefit of their students, junior surgical colleagues, peers, and patients. To them, I owe much gratitude for their cooperation, advice, intellect, experience, wise counsel, friendship and help, for their time, and for their continued encouragement in this rather long-term and complex project. I have already used the text material myself with good effect and it has helped me enormously in my surgical practice.

The text aims to provide health professionals with useful information, which can be selectively used to better inform patients of the potential surgical complications, risks and consequences. I sincerely hope it fulfils this role.

Adelaide, SA, Australia   Brendon J. Coventry, BMBS, PhD,
                                                                            FRACS, FACS, FRSM

Acknowledgements

I wish to thank:

The many learned friends and experienced colleagues who have contributed in innumerable ways along the way in the writing of this text.

Professor Sir Peter Morris, formerly Professor of Surgery at Oxford University, and also Past-President of the College of Surgeons of England, for allowing me to base my initial work at the Nuffield Department of Surgery (NDS) and John Radcliffe Hospital in the University of Oxford, for the UK sector of the studies. He and his colleagues have provided encouragement and valuable discussion time over the course of the project.

The (late) Professor John Farndon, Professor of Surgery at the University of Bristol, Bristol Royal Infirmary, UK; and Professor Robert Mansel, Professor of Surgery at the University of Wales, Cardiff, UK for discussions and valued advice.

Professor Charles Balch, then Professor of Surgery at the Johns Hopkins University, Baltimore, Maryland, USA, and Professor Clifford Ko, from UCLA and American College of Surgeons NSQIP Program, USA, for helpful discussions.

Professor Armando Guiliano, formerly of the John Wayne Cancer Institute, Santa Monica, California, USA for his contributions and valuable discussions.

Professor Jonathan Meakins, then Professor of Surgery at McGill University, Quebec, Canada, who provided helpful discussions and encouragement, during our respective sabbatical periods, which coincided in Oxford; and later as Professor of Surgery at Oxford University.

Over the last decade, numerous clinicians have discussed and generously contributed their experience to the validation of the range and relative frequency of complications associated with the wide spectrum of surgical procedures. These clinicians include:

Los Angeles, USA: Professor Carmack Holmes, Cardiothoracic Surgeon, Los Angeles (UCLA); Professor Donald Morton, Melanoma Surgeon, Los Angeles; Dr R Essner, Melanoma Surgeon, Los Angeles.

New York, USA: Professor Murray Brennan; Dr David Jacques; Prof L Blumgart; Dr Dan Coit; Dr Mary Sue Brady (Surgeons, Department of Surgery, Memorial Sloan-Kettering Cancer Centre, New York);

Oxford, UK: Dr Linda Hands, Vascular Surgeon; Dr Jack Collin, Vascular Surgeon; Professor Peter Friend, Transplant and Vascular Surgeon; Dr Nick Maynard, Upper Gastrointestinal Surgeon; Dr Mike Greenall, Breast Surgeon; Dr Jane Clark, Breast Surgeon; Professor Derek Gray, Vascular/Pancreatic Surgeon; Dr Julian Britton, Hepato-Biliary Surgeon; Dr Greg Sadler, Endocrine Surgeon; Dr Christopher Cunningham, Colorectal Surgeon; Professor Neil Mortensen, Colorectal Surgeon; Dr Bruce George, Colorectal Surgeon; Dr Chris Glynn, Anaesthetist (National Health Service (NHS), Oxford, UK).

Bristol, UK: Professor Derek Alderson.

Adelaide, Australia: Professor Guy Ludbrook, Anesthetist; Dr Elizabeth Tam, Anesthetist.

A number of senior medical students at the University of Adelaide, including Hwee Sim Tan, Adelaine S Lam, Ramon Pathi, Mohd Azizan Ghzali, William Cheng, Sue Min Ooi, Teena Silakong, and Balaji Rajacopalin, who assisted during their student projects in the preliminary feasibility studies and research, and their participation is much appreciated. Thanks also to numerous sixth year students, residents and surgeons at Hospitals in Adelaide who participated in questionnaires and surveys.

The support of the University of Adelaide, especially the Department of Surgery, and Royal Adelaide Hospital has been invaluable in allowing the sabbatical time to engineer the collaborations necessary for this project to progress. I thank Professors Glyn Jamieson and Guy Maddern for their support in this regard.

I especially thank the Royal Australasian College of Surgeons for part-support through the Marjorie Hooper Fellowship.

I thank my clinical colleagues on the Breast, Endocrine and Surgical Oncology Unit at the Royal Adelaide Hospital, especially Grantley Gill, James Kollias and Melissa Bochner, for caring for my patients and assuming greater clinical load when I have been away.

Professor Bill Runciman, Australian Patient Safety Foundation, for all of his advice and support; Professors Cliff Hughes and Bruce Barraclough, from the Royal Australasian College of Surgeons, the Clinical Excellence Commission, New South Wales, and the Australian Commission (Council) on Safety and Quality in Healthcare.

Thanks too to Kai Holt, Anne-Marie Bennett and Carrie Cooper who assisted and helped to organise my work. I also acknowledge my collaborator Martin Ashdown for being so patient during distractions from our scientific research work. Also to Graeme Cogdell, Imagart Design Ltd, Adelaide, for his expertise and helpful discussions.

I particularly thank Melissa Morton and her global team at Springer-Verlag for their work in preparing the manuscript for publication.

Importantly, I truly appreciate and thank my wife Christine, my four children and our parents/ wider family for their support in every way towards seeing this project through to its completion, and in believing so much in me, and in my work.

Adelaide, SA, Australia   Brendon J. Coventry, BMBS, PhD,
                                                                              FRACS, FACS, FRSM

Contents

Contributors

Felix C. Behan, FRCS, FRACS Plastic, Reconstructive and Hand Surgery Unit, University of Melbourne, Western Hospital, Footscray, VIC, Australia

Brendon J. Coventry, BMBS, PhD, FRACS, FACS, FRSM Discipline of Surgery, Royal Adelaide Hospital, University of Adelaide, Adelaide, SA, Australia

A. Gerson Greenburg, MD, PhD The Miriam Hospital, Providence, RI, USA

Department of General Surgery, Brown University Medical School, Providence, RI, USA

William McCarthy, AM, MBBS, FRACS, MEd University of Sydney, Sydney, NSW, Australia

Sydney Melanoma Unit, Royal Prince Alfred Hospital, Camperdown, NSW, Australia

R. Gwyn Morgan, MBBS, FRACS Flinders Medical Centre, Adelaide, SA, Australia

Christopher O'Brien, MS, MD, FRCS (HON), FRACS (Deceased) Sydney Head and Neck Cancer Institute, Sydney, NSW, Australia

Svante R. Orell, ML(Stockholm), FRCPA, FIAC Clinpath Laboratories, Kent Town, SA, Australia

Guy Rees, MBBS, FRACS University of Adelaide, Adelaide, SA, Australia

Royal Adelaide Hospital, Adelaide, SA, Australia

Peter Stavrou, MBBS, FRACS, FA, Ortho A University of Adelaide, Royal Adelaide Hospital, Adelaide, SA, Australia

Chapter 1
Introduction

Brendon J. Coventry

This volume deals with complications, risks, and consequences related to a range of procedures under the broad headings of diagnostic biopsies, cutaneous surgery, including wound closures, skin flaps and grafts, more specific surgical procedures of the hand and foot, hernia surgery, and, finally, a range of relatively commonly performed procedures of the head and neck.

IMPORTANT NOTE: It should be emphasized that the risks and frequencies that are given here *represent derived figures.* These *figures are best estimates of relative frequencies across most institutions,* not merely the highest-performing ones, and as such are often representative of a number of studies, which include different patients with differing comorbidities and different surgeons. In addition, the risks of complications in lower or higher risk patients may lie outside these estimated ranges, and individual clinical judgment is required as to the expected risks communicated to the patient, staff, or for other purposes. The range of risks is also derived from experience and the literature; while risks outside this range may exist, certain risks may be reduced or absent due to variations of procedures or surgical approaches. It is recognized that different patients, practitioners, institutions, regions, and countries may vary in their requirements and recommendations.

Individual clinical judgment should always be exercised, of course, when applying the general information contained in these documents to individual patients in a clinical setting.

Acknowledgments The authors would like to thank and acknowledge the following experienced clinician who discussed the chapters and acted as an advisor: Professor Jonathan Meakins, Montreal, Canada, and Oxford, UK.

B.J. Coventry, BMBS, PhD, FRACS, FACS, FRSM
Discipline of Surgery, Royal Adelaide Hospital, University of Adelaide,
L5 Eleanor Harrald Building, North Terrace,
5000 Adelaide, SA, Australia
e-mail: brendon.coventry@adelaide.edu.au

B.J. Coventry (ed.), *Peripheral, Head and Neck Surgery,*
Surgery: Complications, Risks and Consequences,
DOI 10.1007/978-1-4471-5415-0_1, © Springer-Verlag London 2014

Chapter 2
Diagnostic Biopsy Procedures

Brendon J. Coventry and Svante R. Orell

General Perspective and Overview:

The relative risks and complications of Fine Needle Aspiration Biopsy (also termed Fine Needle Biopsy or Fine Needle Aspiration Cytology/ FNAC) (FNAB) or core needle biopsy (CNB) increase proportionately according to the site of needle biopsy, extent of procedure performed, technique, guidance (if needed), and the needle size. Large bore needle biopsies of highly vascular tissues carry higher risk of bleeding than less vascular structures. Similarly, risk is relatively higher for larger bore needle biopsies performed closer to neural structures (e.g., facial nerve).

Close cooperation is particularly helpful between the pathologist and the surgeon, and if the FNAB or core biopsy is radiologically guided or needs to be selectively sampled, then close involvement of the radiologist is important to have the highest probability of a satisfactory sample for diagnostic purposes. The pathology laboratory staff or pathologist may also advise on the optimal preparation methods, for example, air-dried versus alcohol fixation.

Possible reduction in the risk of misunderstandings over complications or consequences from fine needle biopsy or CNB might be achieved by:

- Good explanation of the risks, aims, benefits, and limitations of the FNAB or CNB procedure
- Careful planning considering the anatomy, approach, alternatives, and method
- Avoiding likely associated vessels and nerves

B.J. Coventry, BMBS, PhD, FRACS, FACS, FRSM (✉)
Discipline of Surgery, Royal Adelaide Hospital, University of Adelaide,
L5 Eleanor Harrald Building, North Terrace,
5000 Adelaide, SA, Australia
e-mail: brendon.coventry@adelaide.edu.au

S.R. Orell, ML(Stockholm), FRCPA, FIAC
Clinpath Laboratories, Kent Town, Adelaide, SA, Australia

B.J. Coventry (ed.), *Peripheral, Head and Neck Surgery*,
Surgery: Complications, Risks and Consequences,
DOI 10.1007/978-1-4471-5415-0_2, © Springer-Verlag London 2014

• Adequate clinical follow-up

With these factors and facts in mind, the information given in this chapter must be appropriately and discernibly interpreted and used.

IMPORTANT NOTE: It should be emphasized that the risks and frequencies that are given here represent derived figures. These are often representative of a number of studies, which include different patients with differing comorbidities. As such, the risks of complications in lower or higher risk patients may lie outside these estimated ranges, and individual clinical judgment is required as to the expected risks communicated to the patient/staff/and for other purposes. The range of risks is also derived from experience and the literature; while risks outside this range may exist, certain risks may be reduced or absent due to certain variations of procedures or surgical approaches. It is recognized that different patients, practitioners, institutions, regions, and countries may vary in their requirements and recommendations.

For diagnostic open biopsies of cutaneous lesions (see chap. 3), or for lymph nodes surgery (see Volume 3), or for other types of biopsies used to obtain diagnosis, refer to the relevant volume and chapter.

Fine Needle (Aspiration) Biopsy

Description

Fine needle aspiration biopsy (FNAB) sampling utilizes a fine-gauge hollow needle (usually 21, 25, or 27 g), usually connected to a syringe. The needle is passed into a mass or lesion several times. Gentle aspiration may be applied using the syringe, or some operators prefer no aspiration, to obtain a specimen of cells within the barrel of the needle, which is then expelled onto a glass slide. The capillary pressure of the needle passing into the mass (often for small target lesions) can often draw sufficient cells into the needle to provide a good sample, without aspiration. Some operators prefer using the needle alone to make multiple passes through the lump, then connect the syringe to expel the contents of the needle. The volume of this latter method is often less, but the quality often higher, with less blood admixed. A smear is usually made across the glass slide using another slide to create a thin layer of cells for cytological assessment. Wet fixation with ethanol spray is sometimes used. Local anesthetic is usually not required, but is sometimes utilized.

Anatomical Points

The characteristics of the mass, lump, or lesion will vary depending on the location and the underlying disease process. Some lesions are not amenable to FNAB. Biopsies within, or close, to lung or pleura may cause a pneumothorax.

Table 2.1 Fine needle aspiration biopsy estimated frequency of complications, risks, and consequences

Complications, risks, and consequences	Estimated frequency
Most significant/serious complications	
Bleeding or haematoma formation[a]	1–5 %
Pain/discomfort/tenderness[a]	20–50 %
Pneumothorax (for trans-thoracic needle biopsy passes)[a]	1–5 %[a]
Rare significant/serious problems	
Neural injury (minor)[a]	0.1–1 %
Neural injury (major)[a]	<0.1 %
Infection[a]	0.1–1 %
Failure to diagnose[a]	0.1–1 %
Spread of malignancy[a]	<0.1 %
Pneumothorax (superficial chest biopsies accidental pleural entry)[a]	<0.1 %
Less serious complications	
Bruising	50–80 %

[a]Depends on underlying pathology, situation, technique preferences, and location in the body

Perspective

Fine needle aspiration biopsy has been used for a number of decades as a useful method of obtaining diagnosis of masses and offers a generally high degree of safety with almost no major side-effects in the vast majority of cases. Pain and discomfort are usually minor, as for a blood sampling (venepuncture) procedure. Discomfort may possibly be lessened with a finer (27 g) needle. Bruising is not unexpected, usually unpredictable and occasionally heralded by a heavily blood stained aspirate. The patient should be warned of the risks shown in Table 2.1, but reassured that the risks are generally minor and usually do not outweigh the diagnostic benefits. There are reports of possible spread of malignant cells with transabdominal puncture of pancreatic masses, but these are largely anecdotal, and an alternative approach can often be used via the postero-lateral muscula-ture, avoiding the transperitoneal route. Transperitoneal FNAB of ovarian masses is discouraged due to the risk of peritoneal seeding. Similar logic may be applied to transperitoneal FNAB of other malignancies. Trans-scrotal FNAB of testicu-lar lesions is also often avoided because of the risk of spread of malignancy across scrotal tissue planes. Failure to diagnose is dependant on many factors, including the site of the mass, the tumor characteristics, operator experience, the sample, the cytologist, and the number of samples taken. Repeated FNAB sam-ples can be performed and this may possibly reduce the risk of a failed diagnosis, but may increase the risk of bleeding. Close clinical follow-up and/or the use of repeated imaging or FNAB with needle guidance using imaging may be helpful.

Major Complications

Major complications are rare, including **nerve injury**, **bleeding**, and **infection**, which are rarely a problem for more than a few days if they should occur. Rare instances of longer-term pain due to nerve injury can occur, but careful anatomical approaches can often reduce this possibility. **Malignant spread** is possible; however, such instances must be rare, as the literature would indicate that local recurrences after FNAB are infrequent if they occur at all. Many subsequent operative approaches incorporate excision of the FNAB site, which is a reason for the FNAB to be performed by the operating surgeon who can plan the definitive surgery. **Failure to diagnose** is a potentially very serious risk using FNAB, but this procedure should be combined with clinical assessment and imaging. It is worth explaining to the patient that FNAB is not always capable of diagnosing with absolute accuracy. False negative and even false positive diagnoses can occur. The level of risk of both failure to diagnose, or spread of malignancy, is determined by many factors, and is given here as an overall guide only. Careful planning, explanation, and follow-up with a cooperative patient approach is often very useful in reducing these risks substantially. **Pneumothorax** is a risk of FNAB performed close to pleura or across/within lung, diaphragm, mediastinal tissues, or at the root of the neck. If risk of pneumothorax is high, admission to hospital for close observation may be wise. The patient should be informed to actively seek the results to avoid **inadequate follow-up**, and to return if the lump changes or enlarges, even if the FNA is not diagnostic, depending on the circumstances.

Consent and Risk Reduction: Fine Needle Aspiration

Main Points to Explain

- Discomfort
- Bruising
- Bleeding
- Perforation (deep biopsies)
- Infection
- Failure to diagnose
- Return for results
- Further procedures/surgery

Core Needle Biopsy

Description

Local anesthetic is usually required. Core needle sampling utilizes a large gauge solid needle (usually 10 g or greater) with a notch in one side connected to a biopsy instrument, often with automatically firing. The needle is passed into a lump and the

Table 2.2 Core needle biopsy estimated frequency of complications, risks, and consequences

Complications, risks, and consequences	Estimated frequency
Most significant/serious complications	
Bleeding/haematoma formation[a] (all)	20–50 %
Major[a]	0.1–1 %
Pain/discomfort/tenderness[a]	20–50 %
Infection[a]	1–5 %
Rare significant/serious problems	
Neural injury (minor)	0.1–1 %
Neural injury (major)	<0.1 %
Dimpling/deformity of the skin	0.1–1 %
Spread of malignancy	<0.1 %
Failure to diagnose	0.1–1 %
Alteration of the subsequent pathology	0.1–1 %
Pneumothorax (superficial chest biopsies accidental pleural entry)[a]	<0.1 %
Less serious complications	
Bruising	>80 %
Scarring	1–5 %

[a]Depends on underlying pathology, surgical technique preferences, and location on the body

sheath automatically advances over the needle to excise a core of tissue. The core sample is then withdrawn for histopathological examination. Approximately a 2 mm diameter cylindrical hole corresponding to the removed core is created, but this tends to collapse aiding hemostasis.

Anatomical Points

The location and consistency of the lump may vary depending on the underlying disease process. Mobile, very deep, or small lumps are often difficult to core sample, as they may be difficult to easily define and secure. Masses close to vascular, neural, or other important structures can increase the risk of complications (Table 2.2).

Perspective

CNB has been used more widely over recent decades as a useful method for obtaining diagnosis of masses and offers a generally high degree of safety with few major known side-effects. Pain and discomfort are usually only moderate, especially with local anesthesia, although considered more than for FNAB. Bruising is frequent, especially when a blood stained sample or leakage occurs. The patient should be warned of the risks above, but reassured that the risks usually do not outweigh the benefits. There are considerations of possible spread of malignant cells, thought due to transection of vessels within the tumor mass. The benefits and risks need to be weighed. As for FNAB, trans-scrotal core biopsy of testicular lesions is also often avoided because of the risk of spread of malignancy across scrotal tissue planes.

Failure to diagnose is dependent on many factors, including the site of the mass, the tumor characteristics, operator experience, the sample, the pathologist, and the number of samples taken. Repeated core biopsy samples can be performed and may possibly reduce the risk of a failed diagnosis. This largely determines the level of risk and frequency. Close clinical follow-up and/or the use of repeated imaging, FNAB or CNB with imaging guidance, may be helpful.

Major Complications

Major complications are rare and **nerve injury**, **bleeding**, and **infection** are rarely a problem for more than a week, if they should occur. The larger needle size increases the risk of side-effects compared with FNAB; however, the diagnostic accuracy is usually improved as pathologists usually prefer CNB samples for diagnosis and the need for an intermediate surgical procedure before definitive surgery may be avoided. Rare instances of longer-term pain due to nerve injury can occur, but careful anatomical approaches or imaging can often reduce this possibility. **Malignant spread** is possible, potentially along the track of the biopsy needle or from transcavity biopsy leakage; however, evidence in the literature is unclear on this issue currently. Many subsequent operative approaches incorporate excision of the core biopsy site, which is a reason for the CNB to be performed by the operating surgeon who can plan the definitive surgery. Failure to diagnose is a potentially very serious risk using CNB, but this procedure should be combined with clinical assessment and imaging. It is worth explaining to the patient that CNB is not always capable of diagnosing with absolute accuracy. The level of risk of both failure to diagnose or spread of malignancy is determined by many factors and is given here as an overall guide only. Careful planning, explanation, and follow-up with a cooperative patient approach are often very useful to reducing these risks substantially. **Pneumothorax** is a risk of CNB performed close to pleura or across/within lung, diaphragm, mediastinal tissues, or at the root of the neck. If risk of pneumothorax or bleeding is high, admission to hospital for close observation may be wise. For this reason it is less commonly used for lung lesion biopsy. The patient should be informed to actively seek the results to avoid **inadequate follow-up**, and to return if the lump changes or enlarges, even if the CNB is not diagnostic, depending on the circumstances.

Consent and Risk Reduction: CNB

Main Points to Explain

- Discomfort
- Bruising
- Bleeding
- Perforation (deep biopsies)

- Infection
- Failure to diagnose
- Return for results
- Further procedures/surgery

Further Reading, References, and Resources

Fine Needle Aspiration

Clemente CD. Anatomy – a regional atlas of the human body. 4th ed. Baltimore: Williams and Wilkins; 1997.

Forsgren L, Orell S. Aspiration cytology in carcinoma of the pancreas. Surgery. 1973;73(1):38–42.

Jamieson GG. The anatomy of general surgical operations. 2nd ed. Edinburgh: Churchill Livingston; 2006.

Knox AM, Fon GT, Orell S. Fine needle aspiration in the chest under CT control. Australas Radiol. 1991;35(2):152–6.

Larsen TE, Little JH, Orell SR, Prade M. International pathologists congruence survey on quantitation of malignant melanoma. Pathology. 1980;12(2):245–53.

Nettle WJ, Orell SR. Fine needle aspiration in the diagnosis of salivary gland lesions. Aust N Z J Surg. 1989;59(1):47–51.

Orell SR. Aspiration cytology in Perth: experience of 673 cases. Med J Aust. 1976;2(5):163–8.

Orell SR. Diagnostic difficulties in the interpretation of fine needle aspirates of salivary gland lesions: the problem revisited. Cytopathology. 1995;6(5):285–300 (review).

Orell SR. Radial scar/complex sclerosing lesion – a problem in the diagnostic work-up of screen-detected breast lesions. Cytopathology. 1999;10(4):250–8.

Orell SR. Pitfalls in fine needle aspiration cytology. Cytopathology. 2003;14(4):173–82 (review).

Orell SR, Farshid G. False-positive reports in fine needle biopsy of breast lesions. Pathology. 2001;33(4):428–36 (review).

Orell SR, Miliauskas J. Fine needle biopsy cytology of breast lesions: a review of interpretative difficulties. Adv Anat Pathol. 2005;12(5):233–45 (review).

Orell SR, Nettle WJ. Fine needle aspiration biopsy of salivary gland tumours. Problems and pitfalls. Pathology. 1988;20(4):332–7.

Orell SR, Philips J. Broadsheet number 57: problems in fine needle biopsy of the thyroid. Pathology. 2000;32(3):191–8 (review).

Orell SR, Langlois SL, Marshall VR. Fine needle aspiration cytology in the diagnosis of solid renal and adrenal masses. Scand J Urol Nephrol. 1985;19(3):211–6.

Orell SR, Sterrett GF, Whitaker D. Fine needle aspiration cytology. 4th ed. Edinburgh: Churchill Livingstone; 2005. ISBN 978-0-443-07364-9.

Whitehead R, Orell S. Biopsy methods in palpable breast lumps. Histopathology. 1979;3(3):247–8.

Core Needle Biopsy

Abe H, Schmidt RA, Kulkarni K, Sennett CA, Mueller JS, Newstead GM. Axillary lymph nodes suspicious for breast cancer metastasis: sampling with US-guided 14-gauge core-needle biopsy – clinical experience in 100 patients. Radiology. 2009;250(1):41–9.

Clemente CD. Anatomy – a regional atlas of the human body. 4th ed. Baltimore: Williams and Wilkins; 1997

Coventry BJ. Core biopsy in preoperative planning of definitive soft-tissue tumour surgery. ANZ J Surg. 2008;78(11):945–6.

Gómez-Rubio M, López-Cano A, Rendón P, Muñoz-Benvenuty A, Macías M, Garre C, Segura-Cabral JM. Safety and diagnostic accuracy of percutaneous ultrasound-guided biopsy of the spleen: a multicenter study. J Clin Ultrasound. 2009;37(8):445–50.

Heyer CM, Reichelt S, Peters SA, Walther JW, Müller KM, Nicolas V. Computed tomography-navigated transthoracic core biopsy of pulmonary lesions: which factors affect diagnostic yield and complication rates? Acad Radiol. 2008;15(8):1017–26.

Jamieson GG. The anatomy of general surgical operations. 2nd ed. Edinburgh: Churchill Livingston; 2006

Khoo TK, Baker CH, Hallanger-Johnson J, Tom AM, Grant CS, Reading CC, Sebo TJ, Morris 3rd JC. Comparison of ultrasound-guided fine-needle aspiration biopsy with core-needle biopsy in the evaluation of thyroid nodules. Endocr Pract. 2008;14(4):426–31.

Laopaiboon V, Aphinives C, Suporntreetriped K. Adequacy and complications of CT-guided percutaneous biopsy: a study of 334 cases in Srinagarind Hospital. J Med Assoc Thai. 2009;92(7):939–46.

Padia SA, Baker ME, Schaeffer CJ, Remer EM, Obuchowski NA, Winans C, Herts BR. Safety and efficacy of sonographic-guided random real-time core needle biopsy of the liver. J Clin Ultrasound. 2009;37(3):138–43.

Soh E, Berman LH, Grant JW, Bullock N, Williams MV. Ultrasound-guided core-needle biopsy of the testis for focal indeterminate intratesticular lesions. Eur Radiol. 2008;18(12):2990–6.

Somerville P, Seifert PJ, Destounis SV, Murphy PF, Young W. Anticoagulation and bleeding risk after core needle biopsy. AJR Am J Roentgenol. 2008;191(4):1194–7.

Steil S, Zerwas S, Moos G, Bittinger F, Hansen T, Mergenthaler U, Weide R. CT-guided percutaneous core needle biopsy in oncology outpatients: sensitivity, specificity, complications. Onkologie. 2009;32(5):254–8.

Thomas T, Kaye PV, Ragunath K, Aithal G. Efficacy, safety, and predictive factors for a positive yield of EUS-guided Trucut biopsy: a large tertiary referral center experience. Am J Gastroenterol. 2009;104(3):584–91.

Volpe A, Mattar K, Finelli A, Kachura JR, Evans AJ, Geddie WR, Jewett MA. Contemporary results of percutaneous biopsy of 100 small renal masses: a single center experience. J Urol. 2008;180(6):2333–7.

Zamboni M, Lannes DC, Cordeiro Pde B, Toscano E, Torquato EB, Cordeiro SS, Cavalcanti A. Transthoracic biopsy with core cutting needle (Trucut) for the diagnosis of mediastinal tumors. Rev Port Pneumol. 2009;15(4):589–95.

Chapter 3
Cutaneous Surgery

Brendon J. Coventry, William McCarthy,
R. Gwyn Morgan, and Felix C. Behan

General Perspective and Overview

The relative risks and complications increase proportionately according to the site of lesion, extent of excision procedure performed, technique, imaging guidance (if needed), and the lesion size. For example, complications overall are more likely in the lower limb because of poorer vascularity. A risk to warn patients of is that of oozing and bleeding which is usually minor and this typically ceases with the application of direct pressure for one or two 20-min intervals. Large excisions in highly vascular tissues carry higher risk of bleeding than for less vascular structures. Risk of numbness and nerve problems are relatively higher for larger and deeper lesion excisions overall, and especially performed closer to neural structures (e.g., peripheral nerves, especially the facial nerve). With regard to scarring, it needs to be explained to the patient that some scarring is usual, but if the lesion is not removed with surgery the consequence may be far more of a problem. In certain body areas, such as the shoulder, sternal region, or upper breast skin, or in regions exposed to

B.J. Coventry, BMBS, PhD, FRACS, FACS, FRSM (✉)
Discipline of Surgery, Royal Adelaide Hospital, University of Adelaide,
L5 Eleanor Harrald Building, North Terrace,
5000 Adelaide, SA, Australia
e-mail: brendon.coventry@adelaide.edu.au

W. McCarthy, AM, MBBS, FRACS, MEd
University of Sydney, Sydney, NSW, Australia

Sydney Melanoma Unit, Royal Prince Alfred Hospital, Camperdown, NSW, Australia

R.G. Morgan, MBBS, FRACS
Flinders Medical Centre, Adelaide, SA, Australia

F.C. Behan, FRCS, FRACS
Plastic & Reconstructive Hand Surgery Unit, University of Melbourne,
Western Hospital, Footscray, Melbourne, VIC, Australia

B.J. Coventry (ed.), *Peripheral, Head and Neck Surgery*,
Surgery: Complications, Risks and Consequences,
DOI 10.1007/978-1-4471-5415-0_3, © Springer-Verlag London 2014

radiotherapy, or with past scarring, hypertrophic or keloid scarring is more common. Flaps and grafts require an explanation of the possibility of partial or total failure, and the need for dressings and/or further surgery. The risks of graft donor site complications also need to be considered in addition to the wound site complications.

Possible reduction in the risk of misunderstandings over complications or consequences from excisions might be achieved by:

- Good explanation of the risks, aims, benefits, and limitations of the procedure
- Useful planning considering the anatomy, approach, alternatives, and method
- Avoiding likely associated vessels and nerves
- Adequate clinical follow-up

With these factors and facts in mind, the information given in this chapter must be appropriately and discernibly interpreted and used.

IMPORTANT NOTE: It should be emphasized that the risks and frequencies that are given here *represent derived figures*. These *figures are best estimates of relative frequencies across most institutions*, not merely the highest-performing ones, and as such are often representative of a number of studies, which include different patients with differing comorbidities and different surgeons. In addition, the risks of complications in lower or higher risk patients may lie outside these estimated ranges, and individual clinical judgment is required as to the expected risks communicated to the patient, staff, or for other purposes. The range of risks is also derived from experience and the literature; while risks outside this range may exist, certain risks may be reduced or absent due to variations of procedures or surgical approaches. It is recognized that different patients, practitioners, institutions, regions, and countries may vary in their requirements and recommendations.

For diagnostic needle biopsies of lesions (Chap. 2) or lymph nodes (see Volume 3), or other biopsies used to obtain diagnosis refer to the relevant volume and chapter.

Surgery for Removal of Skin Lesions

Description

Local anesthetic is usually used or occasionally general anesthetic is required, especially for children, for some facial lesions or for deep and large lesions. The aim is to remove the entire skin lesion with a margin of normal tissue to reduce the risk of possible recurrence. A simple elliptical incision is often used. The wound is usually closed with simple skin suture. Histopathological examination is then performed.

Anatomical Points

The location, type, and appearance of skin lesion often vary widely and treatment options will also depend on the body region and type of lesion to be removed.

Table 3.1 Surgery for removal of skin lesions estimated frequency of complications, risks, and consequences

Complications, risks, and consequences	Estimated frequency
Most significant/serious complications	
Bleeding or hematoma formation[a]	1–5 %
Infection[a]	1–5 %
Hypertrophic/keloidal scarring[a] (overall)	1–5 %
Special body sites (e.g., sternum, shoulder)[a]	5–20 %
Requirement for possible further excision[a]	1–5 %
Rare significant/serious problems	
Numbness and nerve problems[a]	0.1–1 %
Dehiscence[a]	0.1–1 %
Tumor recurrence[a]	Individual
Need for skin flaps or grafts[a]	Individual
Less serious complications	
Pain/discomfort/tenderness[a]	1–5 %
Bruising	1–5 %
Scarring	5–20 %
Dimpling/deformity of the skin/poor cosmesis[a]	1–5 %
Drain tube(s)	<0.1 %

[a]Depends on underlying pathology, surgical technique preferences and location on the body

Excessively fixed, very deeply invasive, large, or ill-defined skin lesions may be difficult to excise, as are those close to vascular or neural structures. Invasion of a nerve by tumor or injury or division of the nerve may occur, partially predicted by location (Table 3.1).

Perspective

The risk of surgery should always be balanced with the benefits. The usual reasons for removal of skin lesions are for malignancy, diagnosis, irritation, discomfort, bleeding, progressive change, or cosmesis. Most complications and consequences are minor. Infection mainly represents an inconvenience of variable importance, but in some people, such as diabetics or immunosuppressed patients, can be life threatening. Cosmetic considerations may be an indication for surgery, but the risk of a non-cosmetic scar is important to discuss prior to surgery, as is the potential for nerve injury (sensory or motor), especially on the face (facial nerve) if deep, or around the eye where retraction can be a problem. Bleeding is rarely a problem, but significant bleeds can occur especially in elderly or anticoagulated patients. Flap or edge necrosis is rarely a problem, but may necessitate further surgery and should be mentioned to the patient, especially in situations of previous radiotherapy to the area.

Major Complications

Major complications are rare; however, **infection** may be local in the wound, with or without **wound dehiscence**, or very rarely become systemic, either with or without **further surgery**. Diabetic, immunosuppressed, or those traveling to remote areas may prompt earlier surgical intervention. Misdiagnosis is a potential problem in some instances with a variety of other cutaneous lesions, and the use of cryotherapy instead of surgery can delay accurate diagnosis, especially for atypical nonpigmented melanomas. A risk to warn patients of is that of **oozing and bleeding** which is usually minor and this typically ceases with application of direct pressure for one or two 20-min intervals. **Nerve injury** is rare overall, but can cause substantial parasthesia or discomfort, especially with, for example, forehead lesions deeply excised. **Wound scarring** with **poor cosmesis** can occur, as can hypertrophic or keloidal scarring. Major complications do not feature the majority of the time.

Consent and Risk Reduction

Main Points to Explain

- Discomfort
- Bruising
- Bleeding
- Infection
- Dehiscence
- Failure to diagnose
- Return for results
- Further procedures/surgery

Surgery for Removal of Cysts, Lipomas, or Other Lumps

Description

Local anesthetic is usually used or occasionally general anesthetic is required, especially for children or for deep, large cysts. The lump may be a sebaceous (epidermoid) or dermoid cyst, a lipoma or another type of cutaneous or subcutaneous lesion. It is usually completely excised with a margin of normal tissue to adequately remove all of the cyst wall or lipoma, without incising into the mass, to reduce the risk of recurrence. The wound is usually closed in layers and the skin sutured. Histopathological examination is then performed.

Table 3.2 Surgery for removal of cysts, lipomas, or other lumps estimated frequency of complications, risks, and consequences

Complications, risks, and consequences	Estimated frequency
Most significant/serious complications	
Bleeding or hematoma formation[a]	1–5 %
Infection[a]	1–5 %
Hypertrophic/keloidal scarring[a]	1–5 %
Special body sites (e.g., sternum, shoulder)[a]	5–20 %
Requirement for possible further excision[a]	1–5 %
Rare significant/serious problems	
Numbness and nerve problems[a]	0.1–1 %
Dehiscence[a]	0.1–1 %
Tumor recurrence[a]	Individual
Cyst recurrence[a]	1–5 %
Need for skin flaps or grafts[a]	Individual
Less serious complications	
Pain/discomfort/tenderness	
Acute (<4 weeks)[a]	20–50 %
Chronic (>12 weeks)[a]	0.1–1 %
Bruising	5–20 %
Scarring	5–20 %
Dimpling/deformity of the skin/poor cosmesis[a]	1–5 %
Drain tube(s)[a]	0.1–1 %

[a]Dependent on underlying pathology, surgical technique preferences, and location on the body

Anatomical Points

The location and consistency of the lump may vary, but is usually over the head, neck, or back regions. Excessively fixed, very deep or ill-defined lumps may be difficult to excise. Lumps close to nerves or vessels present danger of injury or division to these structures. Occasionally, lipomas may insinuate between muscle groups, nerves, and other structures, increasing operative difficulty. Dermoid cysts may (embryologically) communicate through the skull with the dura (external angular dermoid cyst) and pose some risk of intracranial infection (Table 3.2).

Perspective

The risk of surgery should always be balanced with the benefits. Inflammation or recurrent infection mainly represent an inconvenience of variable importance, but in some people, such as diabetics or immunosuppressed patients, can be life threatening. Cosmetic considerations may be an indication for surgery, but the risk of a non-cosmetic scar, especially in situations of previous radiotherapy to the area, is important to discuss prior to surgery, as is the potential for nerve injury (sensory or motor). Postoperative infection is useful to consider versus the risk of recurrent infections of the cyst without surgery. Many cysts never become inflamed or infected, while others incur repeated inflammation, although both are often unpredictable. The size and location of the cyst may dictate the need for drain tubes, and the effects of scarring or poor cosmesis, especially in situations of previous radiotherapy to the area.

Major Complications

Major complications are rare; however, **infection** may be local in the wound, with or without **wound dehiscence**, or very rarely become systemic, either with or without **further surgery**. The risk of infection postoperatively is often reduced by treating an active infection with appropriate antibiotic therapy for 2–3 weeks prior to surgery to settle the infection. Diabetic, immunosuppressed, or those traveling to remote areas may prompt earlier surgical intervention. A risk to warn patients of is that of **oozing and bleeding** which is usually minor and this typically ceases with application of direct pressure for one or two 20-min intervals. **Misdiagnosis** is a potential problem in some instances with a variety of other subcutaneous lesions that may mimic a sebaceous cyst, most notably metastatic melanoma. Imaging and needle cytology may assist where appropriate, for uncertain lesions, to reduce the risk from inappropriate surgery that may possibly jeopardize the outcome. However, this considered, the usual clinical diagnostic history and signs of a sebaceous cyst are correct the majority of the time. **Nerve injury** is rare, but can cause substantial parasthesia or discomfort. **Wound scarring** with **poor cosmesis** can occur, as can hypertrophic or keloidal scarring. Major complications do not feature the majority of the time.

Consent and Risk Reduction

Main Points to Explain

- Discomfort
- Bruising
- Bleeding
- Infection
- Dehiscence
- Possible recurrence
- Failure to diagnose
- Return for results
- Further procedures/surgery

Surgery for Wide Local Excision

Description

General anesthetic or local anesthetic is used. The aim is to excise a margin of normal skin around a melanoma site to reduce risk of local recurrence. The margin will depend on location on the body and tumor thickness. Fascia may need to be included in the excision as may superficial veins, arteries, or nerves. Primary closure is usually performed, but flap repair or grafting may be required. The procedure may be combined with sentinel node biopsy. Histopathological examination is then performed.

Anatomical Points

The site where the excision is being performed will dictate the ease or difficulty of wide local excision (WLE). Lesions on the nose, eyelids, ears, face, genitals, distal limbs, or in the oral cavity or anus are more complex to obtain an adequate margin than lesions where more skin is available, such as abdomen and back. The presence of nerves and other vital structures adds complexity since these may be injured or need to be sacrificed (Table 3.3).

Table 3.3 Surgery for wide local excision (WLE) estimated frequency of complications, risks, and consequences

Complications, risks, and consequences	Estimated frequency
Most significant/serious complications	
Bleeding or hematoma formation[a]	5–20 %
Infection[a]	1–5 %
Hypertrophic/keloidal scarring[a]	1–5 %
Special body sites (e.g., sternum, shoulder)[a]	5–20 %
Requirement for possible further excision[a]	1–5 %
Rare significant/serious problems	
Edge/flap necrosis	0.1–1 %
Numbness and nerve problems[a]	1–5 %
Wound dehiscence[a]	0.1–1 %
Tumor recurrence[a]	Individual
Need for skin flaps or grafts[a]	Individual
Loss of skin graft (partial or complete)[a]	1–5 %
Less serious complications	
Pain/discomfort/tenderness	
Acute (<4 weeks)[a]	20–50 %
Chronic (>12 weeks)[a]	0.1–1 %
Bruising	20–50 %
Scarring	5–20 %
Reduced mobility (short term)[a]	5–20 %
Dimpling/deformity of the skin/poor cosmesis[a]	1–5 %
Drain tube(s)[a]	1–5 %

[a]Dependent on underlying pathology, surgical technique preferences and location on the body

Perspective

The risk of surgery should always be balanced with the benefits. The usual reason for wider excision of skin around a melanoma site is to reduce risk of recurrence. Most complications and consequences are relatively minor. Infection mainly represents an inconvenience of variable importance, but in some people, such as diabetics or immunosuppressed patients, can be life threatening. The risk of a non-cosmetic scar is important to discuss prior to surgery, especially in situations of previous radiotherapy to the area, as is the potential for nerve injury (sensory or motor), especially on the face (facial nerve) if deep, or around the eye where retraction can be a problem. Bleeding is rarely a problem, but significant bleeds can occur especially in elderly or anticoagulated patients. Flap or edge necrosis is rarely a problem, but may necessitate further surgery and should be mentioned to the patient, especially in situations of previous radiotherapy to the area. Skin graft loss is more likely in the lower limb because of poorer vascularity.

Major Complications

Major complications are rare; however, **infection** may be local in the wound, with or without **wound dehiscence**, or very rarely become systemic, either with or without **further surgery**. The risk of infection postoperatively is often reduced by treating an active infection with appropriate antibiotic therapy for 2–3 weeks prior to surgery to settle the infection. Diabetic, immunosuppressed, or those traveling to remote areas may prompt earlier surgical intervention. **Inadequate margins** of excision are a potential problem and may require **further surgery**. Despite performing a WLE, **tumor recurrence** is an important risk to warn patients of, but this is more determined by tumor biology. **Nerve injury** is rare, but can cause substantial parasthesia or discomfort and be a significant issue. **Wound scarring** with **poor cosmesis** can occur, as can hypertrophic or keloidal scarring. The most major risk to warn patients of is that of **oozing and bleeding** which is usually minor and this typically ceases with application of direct pressure for one or two 20-min intervals. **Total flap necrosis** is very rare, but should be mentioned because it will often require prolonged dressings or further surgery. Major complications do not feature the majority of the time.

Consent and Risk Reduction

Main Points to Explain

- Discomfort
- Bruising
- Bleeding

- Infection
- Dehiscence
- Possible recurrence
- Failure to diagnose
- Return for results
- Further procedures/surgery

Small or Simple Local Skin Flap Repair Surgery

Description

Local anesthetic is usually used or occasionally general anesthetic is required, especially for children, some facial lesions or for deep, large lesions, and/or flaps. The aim is to provide a means of using surrounding skin to primarily close a defect with skin sutures, usually after removal of a skin lesion. Histopathological examination is then typically performed on any lesion removed.

Anatomical Points

The location, type, construction, ease, and appearance of skin flap can vary widely depending on the body region and type of lesion to be removed. Large, deep, or complex flap repairs may involve vascular or neural structures. Division of the nerve may occur, partially predicted by location (Table 3.4).

Perspective

The risk of surgery should always be balanced with the benefits. The usual reason for flap repair is to provide easier primary closure, usually with improved cosmesis. Most complications and consequences are relatively minor. Infection mainly represents an inconvenience of variable importance, but in some people, such as diabetics or immunosuppressed patients, can be life threatening. The risk of a non-cosmetic scar is important to discuss prior to surgery, as is the potential for nerve injury (sensory or motor), especially on the face (facial nerve) if deep, or around the eye where retraction can be a problem. Bleeding is rarely a problem, but significant bleeds can occur especially in elderly or anticoagulated patients. Flap or edge necrosis is rarely a problem, but may necessitate further surgery and should be mentioned to the patient, especially in situations of previous radiotherapy to the area. Complication overall are more likely in the lower limb because of poorer vascularity.

Table 3.4 Small or simple local skin flaps estimated frequency of complications, risks, and consequences

Complications, risks, and consequences	Estimated frequency
Most significant/serious complications	
Bleeding or hematoma formation[a]	5–20 %
Infection[a]	1–5 %
Hypertrophic/keloidal scarring[a]	1–5 %
Special body sites (e.g., sternum, shoulder)[a]	5–20 %
Requirement for possible further excision[a]	1–5 %
Necrosis of wound edges[a]	
Flap tip necrosis	1–5 %
Total flap failure	0.1–1 %
Rare significant/serious problems	
Wound dehiscence[a]	0.1–1 %
Tumor recurrence[a]	Individual
Cyst recurrence[a]	1–5 %
Necessity for further skin flaps or grafts[a]	<0.1 %
Less serious complications	
Pain/discomfort/tenderness	
Acute (<4 weeks)[a]	20–50 %
Chronic (>12 weeks)[a]	0.1–1 %
Numbness and nerve problems[a]	1–5 %
Bruising	20–50 %
Scarring	5–20 %
Reduced mobility (short term)[a]	5–20 %
Dimpling/deformity of the skin/poor cosmesis[a]	1–5 %
Drain tube(s)[a]	0.1–1 %

[a]Dependent on underlying pathology, surgical technique preferences, and location on the body

Major Complications

Major complications are rare; however, **infection** may be local in the wound, with or without **wound dehiscence**, or very rarely become systemic, either with or without **further surgery**. The risk of infection postoperatively is often reduced by treating an active infection with appropriate antibiotic therapy for 2–3 weeks prior to surgery to settle the infection. Diabetic, immunosuppressed, or those traveling to remote areas may prompt earlier surgical intervention. **Inadequate margins** of excision are a potential problem and may require **further surgery**. **Nerve injury** is rare, but can cause substantial parasthesia or discomfort. **Wound scarring** with **poor cosmesis** can occur, as can hypertrophic or keloidal scarring. The most major risk to warn patients of is that of **oozing and bleeding** which is usually minor and this typically ceases with application of direct pressure for one or two 20-min intervals. **Total flap necrosis** is very rare, but should be mentioned because it will often require prolonged dressings or further surgery. Major complications do not feature the majority of the time.

Consent and Risk Reduction

Main Points to Explain

- Discomfort
- Bruising
- Bleeding
- Infection
- Dehiscence
- Graft loss (partial or total)
- Possible recurrence
- Failure to diagnose
- Return for results
- Further procedures/surgery

Complex or Large Skin Flap Repair Surgery

Description

Local anesthetic is usually used or occasionally general anesthetic is required, especially for children, some facial lesions or for deep, large lesions, and/or flaps. The aim is to provide a means of using surrounding skin to primarily close a defect with skin sutures, usually after removal of a skin lesion. Histopathological examination is then typically performed on any lesion removed.

Anatomical Points

The location, type, construction, ease, and appearance of skin flap can vary widely depending on the body region and type of lesion to be removed. Large, deep, or complex flap repairs may involve vascular or neural structures. Division of the nerve may occur, partially predicted by location (Table 3.5).

Perspective

The risk of surgery should always be balanced with the benefits. The risks of complex flap repair are similar, but slightly higher than for simple flaps, being determined by the individual situation. The usual reason for complex flap repair is to provide primary closure, usually with improved cosmesis. Most complications and consequences

Table 3.5 Complex or large skin flap surgery estimated frequency of complications, risks, and consequences

Complications, risks, and consequences	Estimated frequency
Most significant/serious complications	
Bleeding or hematoma formation[a]	5–20 %
Infection[a]	1–5 %
Hypertrophic/keloidal scarring[a]	1–5 %
Special body sites (e.g., sternum, shoulder)[a]	5–20 %
Requirement for possible further excision[a]	1–5 %
Necrosis of wound edges[a]	
Flap tip necrosis	5–20 %
Total flap failure	1–5 %
Cyst recurrence[a]	1–5 %
Necessity for further surgery, skin flaps, or grafts[a]	1–5 %
Wound dehiscence[a]	1–5 %
Rare significant/serious problems	
Tumor recurrence[a]	Individual
Less serious complications	
Pain/discomfort/tenderness	
Acute (<4 weeks)[a]	20–50 %
Chronic (>12 weeks)[a]	0.1–1 %
Numbness and nerve problems[a]	5–20 %
Bruising	>80 %
Scarring	5–20 %
Reduced mobility (short term)[a]	5–20 %
Dimpling/deformity of the skin/poor cosmesis[a]	1–5 %
Drain tube(s)[a]	1–5 %

[a]Dependent on underlying pathology, surgical technique preferences, and location on the body

are relatively minor. Infection mainly represents an inconvenience of variable importance, but in some people, such as diabetics or immunosuppressed patients, can be life threatening. The risk of a non-cosmetic scar is important to discuss prior to surgery, as is the potential for nerve injury (sensory or motor), especially on the face (facial nerve) if deep, or around the eye where retraction can be a problem. Bleeding is rarely a problem, but significant bleeds can occur especially in elderly or anticoagulated patients. Flap or edge necrosis can be a problem, necessitating further surgery and should be mentioned to the patient, especially in situations of previous radiotherapy to the area. Minor flap necrosis is naturally more frequent than with simple flap repair, due to the complex design. Total flap necrosis is rare, but should be mentioned because it will often require prolonged dressings or further surgery.

Major Complications

Major complications are rare; however, **infection** may be local in the wound, with or without **wound dehiscence**, or very rarely become systemic, either with or without **further surgery**. The risk of infection postoperatively is often reduced by treating an active infection with appropriate antibiotic therapy for 2–3 weeks prior to surgery to settle the infection. Diabetic, immunosuppressed, or those traveling to remote areas may prompt earlier surgical intervention. **Inadequate margins** of excision are a potential problem and may require **further surgery**. **Nerve injury** is rare, but can cause substantial parasthesia or discomfort. **Wound scarring** with **poor cosmesis** can occur, as can hypertrophic or keloidal scarring. The most major risk to warn patients of is that of **oozing and bleeding** which is usually minor and this typically ceases with application of direct pressure for one or two 20-min intervals. **Total flap necrosis** is very rare, but **partial flap loss** or **dehiscence** should be mentioned because it will often require prolonged dressings or further surgery. Major complications do not feature the majority of the time.

Consent and Risk Reduction

Main Points to Explain

- Discomfort
- Bruising
- Bleeding
- Infection
- Dehiscence
- Possible recurrence
- Flap loss (partial or total)
- Return for results
- Further procedures/surgery

Island Skin Flap Repair Surgery

Description

Local anesthetic is usually used for smaller flaps, but general anesthetic is usually required for larger flaps, complex flaps, or for children, some facial lesions or for deep, large lesions. The aim is to provide a means of using an island of surrounding skin to primarily close a defect with skin sutures, usually after removal of a skin lesion, or to cover skin loss/ulceration. Histopathological examination is then typically performed on any lesion or abnormal tissues removed. Several types of island flaps are available to construct, typically comprising skin and subcutaneous tissues—cutaneous island flaps, but may include muscle and fascia as well—so-called myocutaneous flap repairs. Keystone island flaps are a form of island flap based primarily on blood supply arising from the deep fascia. There is increasing evidence that augmentation of the deep facial blood supply occurs as a result "sympathectomy" from division of sympathetic nerves traveling with the peripheral vessels that initially supplied the island flap which are divided in the course of formation of the "island."

Anatomical Points

The location, type, construction, ease, and appearance of island skin flap can vary widely depending on the body region and type of lesion to be removed. Large, deep, or complex island flap repairs may involve vascular or neural structures. Division of the nerves may occur, partially predicted by location (Table 3.6).

Perspective

Almost paradoxically island flap repairs are associated with a surprising lack of complications, which may be a result of effective "sympathectomy" of small

Table 3.6 Island skin flap repair surgery estimated frequency of complications, risks, and consequences

Complications, risks, and consequences	Estimated frequency
Most significant/serious complications	
Bleeding or hematoma formation[a]	5–20 %
Infection[a]	1–5 %
Hypertrophic/keloidal scarring[a]	1–5 %
Special body sites (e.g., sternum, shoulder)[a]	5–20 %
Requirement for possible further excision[a]	1–5 %
Necrosis of wound edges[a]	
Flap tip necrosis	5–20 %
Total flap failure	1–5 %
Cyst recurrence[a]	1–5 %
Necessity for further surgery, skin flaps, or grafts[a]	1–5 %
Wound dehiscence[a]	1–5 %
Rare significant/serious problems	
Tumor recurrence[a]	Individual
Less serious complications	
Pain/discomfort/tenderness	
Acute (<4 weeks)[a]	20–50 %
Chronic (>12 weeks)[a]	0.1–1 %
Numbness and nerve problems[a]	5–20 %
Bruising	>80 %
Scarring	5–20 %
Reduced mobility (short term)[a]	5–20 %
Dimpling/deformity of the skin/poor cosmesis[a]	1–5 %
Drain tube(s)[a]	1–5 %

[a]Dependent on underlying pathology, surgical technique preferences, and location on the body

perivascular nerves traveling with the peripheral supplying vessels divided in the course of formation of the "island"—causing relative augmentation of the remaining deep facial blood supply—coined the "Immediate Vascular Augmentation Concept" (IVAC). The risk of surgery should always be balanced with the benefits. The risks of island flap repair are similar, but slightly higher than for simple flaps, being determined by the individual situation and flap complexity. The usual reason for island flap repair is to provide primary closure, usually with improved cosmesis. Most complications and consequences are relatively minor. Infection mainly represents an inconvenience of variable importance, but in some people, such as diabetics or immunosuppressed patients, can be life threatening. The risk of a non-cosmetic scar is important to discuss prior to surgery, as is the potential for nerve injury (sensory or motor), especially on the face (facial nerve) if deep, or around the eye where retraction can be a problem. Bleeding is rarely a problem, but significant bleeds can occur especially in elderly or anticoagulated patients. Flap or edge necrosis can be a problem, necessitating further surgery and should be mentioned to the patient, especially in situations of previous radiotherapy to the area; however, the relative risk of flap necrosis appears less than for other non-island flaps.

Major Complications

Major complications are rare; however, **infection** may be local in the wound, with or without **wound dehiscence**, or very rarely become systemic, either with or without **further surgery**. The risk of infection postoperatively is often reduced by treating an active infection with appropriate antibiotic therapy for 2–3 weeks prior to surgery to settle the infection. Diabetic, immunosuppressed, or those traveling to remote areas may prompt earlier surgical intervention. **Inadequate margins** of excision are a potential problem and may require **further surgery**. **Nerve injury** is rare, but can cause substantial parasthesia or discomfort. **Wound scarring** with **poor cosmesis** can occur, as can hypertrophic or keloidal scarring. The most major risk to warn patients of is that of **oozing and bleeding** which is usually minor and this typically ceases with application of direct pressure for one or two 20-min intervals. **Total flap necrosis** is very rare, but **partial flap loss** or **dehiscence** should be mentioned because it will often require prolonged dressings or further surgery. Major complications do not feature the majority of the time.

Consent and Risk Reduction

Main Points to Explain

- Discomfort
- Bruising
- Bleeding

- Infection
- Dehiscence
- Possible recurrence
- Flap loss (partial or total)
- Return for results
- Further procedures/surgery

Skin Graft Surgery (Split or Full Thickness Grafting)

Description

Local anesthetic is usually used or occasionally general anesthetic is required, especially for children, some facial lesions or for deep, large lesions, and/or flaps. The aim is to provide a means of using transplanted autologous skin to close a defect, often following excision of a skin lesion. Histopathological examination is then typically performed on any lesion removed. Split skin grafts incorporate upper- or mid-dermis, whereas full thickness grafts use all skin layers.

Anatomical Points

The location, type, size, construction, ease, and appearance of skin graft can vary widely depending on the body region and type of lesion to be removed. Large, deep, or invasive lesions may involve vascular or neural structures, or tendons. Division of a nerve may occur, partially predicted by location (Table 3.7).

Perspective

Larger grafts are usually associated with a greater frequency of risks. The risk of surgery should always be balanced with the benefits. The risks of grafting are determined by the individual situation, including the body site, type of graft, underlying condition(s), and size of graft. The usual reason for skin graft repair is to provide closure, usually where primary closure is not feasible. Most complications and consequences are relatively minor. Infection mainly represents an inconvenience of variable importance, but in some people, such as diabetics or immunosuppressed patients, can be life threatening. The risk of a non-cosmetic graft is important to discuss prior to surgery, especially in situations of previous radiotherapy to the area, as is the potential for nerve injury (sensory or motor), especially on the face (facial nerve) if deep, or around the eye where retraction can be a problem. Bleeding is

Table 3.7 Skin graft surgery (split or full thickness grafting) estimated frequency of complications, risks, and consequences

Complications, risks, and consequences	Estimated frequency
Most significant/serious complications	
Bleeding, oozing, or hematoma formation[a]	5–20 %
Infection (donor or graft sites)[a]	5–20 %
Hypertrophic/keloidal scarring[a]	1–5 %
Special body sites (e.g., sternum, shoulder)[a]	5–20 %
Requirement for possible further excision[a]	1–5 %
Necrosis of graft[a]	
Partial necrosis	5–20 %
Total failure	1–5 %
Cyst recurrence[a]	1–5 %
Necessity for further surgery, skin flaps, or grafts[a]	1–5 %
Wound/graft edge dehiscence[a]	1–5 %
Rare significant/serious problems	
Tumor recurrence[a]	Individual
Less serious complications	
Pain/discomfort/tenderness	
Acute (<4 weeks)[a]	20–50 %
Chronic (>12 weeks)[a]	0.1–1 %
Numbness and nerve problems	1–5 %
Bruising	5–20 %
Reduced mobility (short term)[a,b]	20–50 %
Wound scarring/indentation/deformity/poor cosmesis of the skin[a]	50–80 %
Hyper-granulation	1–5 %
Donor site scarring/irritation (long term >6 months)[a]	0.1–1 %
Drain tube(s)[a]	1–5 %

[a]Depends on underlying pathology, surgical technique preferences, skin type, and location on the body
[b]Higher frequency (>80 %) with lower limb grafts and larger grafts

rarely a problem, but significant bleeds can occur especially in elderly or anticoagulated patients. Graft necrosis can be a problem, necessitating further surgery, including re-grafting, and should be mentioned to the patient, again especially in situations of previous radiotherapy to the area.

Major Complications

Major complications are rare; however, **infection** may be local in the wound, with or without **partial or total graft loss** or **wound dehiscence**, or very rarely become systemic, either with or without **further surgery**. An additional risk is **infection of the donor site**. The risk of infection postoperatively may often be reduced by treating an active infection with appropriate antibiotic therapy for 2–3 weeks prior to surgery, to settle the infection. Diabetic, immunosuppressed, or those traveling to remote areas may prompt earlier surgical intervention. **Inadequate margins** of excision are a potential problem and may require **further surgery**. **Nerve injury** is rare, but can cause substantial parasthesia or discomfort. **Wound scarring** with **poor cosmesis** can occur, as can hypertrophic or keloidal scarring. The most major risk to warn patients of is that of **oozing and bleeding** which is usually minor and this typically ceases with application of direct pressure for one or two 20-min intervals. **Total graft necrosis** is very rare, but **partial graft loss** or graft edge **dehiscence** should be mentioned because it is not uncommon and unpredictable, often requiring prolonged dressings or further surgery. Immobilizing the patient using a back slab splint and a short period of bed rest usually with elevation can reduce activity of the (especially lower) limb graft site, reduce risks, and improve outcome. Major complications do not feature the majority of the time.

Consent and Risk Reduction

Main Points to Explain

- Discomfort
- Bruising
- Bleeding
- Infection
- Donor site complications
- Dehiscence
- Graft loss (partial or total)
- Possible recurrence
- Return for results
- Further procedures/surgery

Further Reading, References, and Resources

Balch CM, Houghton AN, Sober AJ, Soong S-J. Cutaneous melanoma. 5th ed. St Louis: Quality Medical Publishing; 2008.

Clemente CD. Anatomy – a regional atlas of the human body. 4th ed. Baltimore: Williams and Wilkins; 1997.

Jamieson GG. The anatomy of general surgical operations. 2nd ed. Edinburgh: Churchill Livingston; 2006.

Thompson JF, Morton DL, Kroon BBR, editors. Textbook of melanoma. London: Martin Dunitz; 2004.

Chapter 4
Hand Surgery

Brendon J. Coventry and R. Gwyn Morgan

General Perspective and Overview

The relative risks and complications increase proportionately according to the type of hand problem, site of lesion/problem, extent of procedure performed, technique, imaging guidance (if needed), and the lesion size. Large excisions in highly vascular tissues carry higher risk of bleeding than for less vascular structures. Advising the patient to keep the hand and arm elevated especially for the 2 weeks after surgery is vital for reducing the risk of bleeding and swelling. Risks of numbness and nerve problems are relatively higher for larger and deeper lesion excisions performed closer to neural structures (e.g., digital nerves). With regard to scarring, it needs to be explained to the patient that some scarring is usual, but if the lesion is not removed with surgery, the consequence may be far more of a problem (depending on the pathology). If necessary, flaps and grafts require an explanation of the possibility of partial or total failure, and the need for dressings and/or further surgery. The risks of graft donor site complications may also need to be considered, in addition to the wound site complications.

Possible reduction in the risk of misunderstandings over complications or consequences from hand surgery might be achieved by:
- Good explanation of the risks, aims, benefits, and limitations of the procedure
- Careful planning considering the anatomy, approach, alternatives, and method
- Avoiding/protecting likely associated vessels and nerves
- Adequate clinical follow-up

B.J. Coventry, BMBS, PhD, FRACS, FACS, FRSM (✉)
Discipline of Surgery, Royal Adelaide Hospital, University of Adelaide,
L5 Eleanor Harrald Building, North Terrace,
5000 Adelaide, SA, Australia
e-mail: brendon.coventry@adelaide.edu.au

R.G. Morgan, MBBS, FRACS
Plastic and Reconstructive Surgeon, Flinders Medical Centre, Adelaide, SA, Australia

B.J. Coventry (ed.), *Peripheral, Head and Neck Surgery,*
Surgery: Complications, Risks and Consequences,
DOI 10.1007/978-1-4471-5415-0_4, © Springer-Verlag London 2014

With these factors and facts in mind, the information given in this chapter must be appropriately and discernibly interpreted and used.

IMPORTANT NOTE: It should be emphasized that the risks and frequencies that are given here *represent derived figures*. These *figures are best estimates of relative frequencies across most institutions*, not merely the highest-performing ones, and as such are often representative of a number of studies, which include different patients with differing comorbidities and different surgeons. In addition, the risks of complications in lower or higher risk patients may lie outside these estimated ranges, and individual clinical judgement is required as to the expected risks communicated to the patient, staff, or for other purposes. The range of risks is also derived from experience and the literature; while risks outside this range may exist, certain risks may be reduced or absent due to variations of procedures or surgical approaches. It is recognized that different patients, practitioners, institutions, regions, and countries may vary in their requirements and recommendations.

For diagnostic needle biopsies of lesions (Chap. 2) or excision of skin lesions (Chap. 3), or other biopsies used to obtain diagnosis, please refer to the relevant volume and chapter.

Surgery for Carpal Tunnel Release (Flexor Retinaculotomy)

Description

Local anesthesia, axillary arm block, ischemic arm block, or general anesthesia can be used. The aim is to release the pressure on the median nerve by longitudinally incising the constricting flexor retinaculum lying across the carpus.

Anatomical Points

The flexor retinaculum is a fibrous ligament that extends from the scaphoid and trapezium on the radial side to the carpus to the triquetral and pisiform on the ulnar side. The flexor retinaculum can extend further into the palm and further into the wrist in some individuals than others. It can also be in more than one part or band. For this reason the entire retinaculum must be divided longitudinally. Persistence of a band of residual retinaculum can fail to relieve the median nerve compression. The flexor retinaculum and/or carpal bones can become thickened, narrowing the carpal tunnel, thereby constricting the median nerve. The palmar branch of the median nerve, which supplies a small area of skin overlying the thenar eminence, lies proximally to the radial side of the flexor retinaculum, but can lie relatively medially. For this reason, the incision is more safely made just to the ulnar side of the median nerve (Table 4.1).

Table 4.1 Surgery for carpal tunnel release (flexor retinaculotomy) estimated frequency of complications, risks, and consequences

Complications, risks, and consequences	Estimated frequency
Most significant/serious complications	
Bleeding or hematoma formation	1–5 %
Infection	1–5 %
Inability to correct long-term symptoms (muscle weakness; anesthesia, or parasthesia)[a] (overall)	1–5 %
For long-standing symptoms[a]	20–50 %
Numbness and nerve problems	1–5 %
Rare significant/serious problems	
Recurrence of symptoms	0.1–1 %
Severe neural injury—median or palmar branch of median nerve	0.1–1 %
Necrosis of skin edges/flaps[a]	0.1–1 %
Reformation of the carpal tunnel[a]	<0.1 %
Necessity for skin flaps or grafts	<0.1 %
Dehiscence	<0.1 %
Less serious complications	
Pain/discomfort/tenderness	
Acute (<2 months)	20–50 %
Chronic (>2 months)	1–5 %
Reduced mobility[a]	
Acute (<2 months)	20–50 %
Chronic (>2 months)	0.1–1 %
Bruising	50–80 %
Wound scarring/deformity (poor cosmesis)	1–5 %

[a]Depending on underlying pathology, state of advancement of disease, surgical technique preferences

Perspective

Surgery for carpal tunnel release is usually very straightforward and complications are few and minor; however, serious complications can be debilitating and necessitate further surgery. Patients should be aware of the small chance of these serious complications. The decision for surgery must be balanced by the risks of the nonoperative alternative of observation and conservative management. However, the presence of significant median nerve entrapment and conduction deficit(s) usually dictates earlier surgical intervention. Infection may be debilitating especially in diabetic or immunosuppressed individuals and occasionally lead to arm cellulitis and even systemic infections. Excessive pressure from bandages or tight sutures from swelling can lead to local necrosis of the wound edges. Bruising due to slow, concealed postoperative bleeding can be spectacular and extend along the tissue plane into the high forearm. Attention to hemostasis during and at the completion of the procedure, and releasing the tourniquet to ensure hemostasis at completion, can reduce the risk of postoperative bleeding.

Major Complications

Bleeding may rarely be severe, causing a concealed palmar hematoma and **re-compressive median nerve symptoms** and can rarely lead to the need for surgical drainage. **Infection,** especially in diabetics or immunosuppressed individuals, may lead to severe limb cellulitis and/or systemic and occasionally life-threatening infection. **Injury to the median nerve** is rarely severe, except when compression has severely damaged the nerve preoperatively. This may cause permanent sensory loss and/or motor deficit, which the patient should be warned about. **Numbness** is otherwise rarely an issue. If infection or necrosis occurs, poor cosmesis can result. **Skin necrosis** and **dehiscence** is rare, but can occur from tight bandaging, or failure to elevate the limb for the first 48–72 h postoperatively due to poor cooperation. **Recurrent median nerve constriction** can occur, necessitating re-operation, but is unusual and unpredictable. Infection of the dominant hand after surgery may significantly impact on function and employment. **Stiffness** can be a significant problem if immobility is prolonged, with **loss of mobility**.

Consent and Risk Reduction

Main Points to Explain

- Discomfort
- Bleeding
- Infection
- Numbness
- Stiffness
- Loss of mobility
- Further surgery

Surgery for Tendovaginitis Stenosans (Trigger Finger) Release

Description

Local anesthesia, axillary arm block, ischemic arm block, or general anesthesia can be used. The aim is to release the constriction of the flexor profundus tendon by longitudinally incising the constricting tunnel of the tendon sheath. This problem

Table 4.2 Surgery for Tendovaginitis stenosans (trigger finger) release estimated frequency of complications, risks, and consequences

Complications, risks, and consequences	Estimated frequency
Most significant/serious complications	
Bleeding or hematoma formation	1–5 %
Infection	1–5 %
Recurrence tendon sheath constriction	1–5 %
Numbness and nerve problems	1–5 %
Rare significant/serious problems	
Severe neural injury—digital nerve	0.1–1 %
Necrosis of skin edges/flaps[a]	0.1–1 %
Necessity for skin flaps or grafts	<0.1 %
Dehiscence	<0.1 %
Less serious complications	
Pain/discomfort/tenderness	
Acute (<2 months)	20–50 %
Chronic (>2 months)	1–5 %
Reduced mobility[a]	
Acute (<2 months)	20–50 %
Chronic (>2 months)	0.1–1 %
Bruising	50–80 %
Wound scarring/deformity (poor cosmesis)	1–5 %
Drain tube(s)[a]	<0.1 %

[a]Depends on underlying pathology, state of advancement of disease, surgical technique preferences

typically involves the ring finger (fourth digit), but other fingers can be involved, especially in diabetics who may have multiple digits involved.

Anatomical Points

The constricting tunnel of the flexor tendon sheath typically lies over the volar aspect of the head of the metacarpal bone of the ring finger. A nodule forms within the tendon proximal to the swollen and narrowed opening of the tendon sheath and "catches" on the narrowed tunnel of the tendon sheath during movement of the tendon/nodule through the sheath, causing a clicking or "trigger" effect. This classically occurs during extension from full flexion as the nodule is pulled through the constricted area of the sheath. Focal pressure over the palm against the metacarpal head from repetitive trauma to the tendon/sheath is thought to produce the nodule and constriction. The site and extent of compression/nodule formation can vary significantly between patients. The digital blood vessels and nerves usually lie more laterally to the median operative longitudinal incision through the constricted area of the sheath (Table 4.2).

Perspective

Surgery for trigger finger release is usually very straightforward and complications are few and minor; however, serious complications can be debilitating and occasionally necessitate further surgery. Patients should be aware of the small chance of these serious complications. The decision for surgery must be balanced by the risks of the non-operative alternative of observation and conservative management. However, the presence of significant finger immobility or discomfort usually dictates earlier surgical intervention. Infection may be debilitating especially in diabetic or immunosuppressed individuals, occasionally leading to arm cellulitis and even systemic infections. Excessive pressure from bandages or tight sutures from swelling can lead to local necrosis of the wound edges. Bruising due to slow, concealed postoperative bleeding can cause hand swelling.

Major Complications

Bleeding may rarely be severe, causing a concealed palmar hematoma can rarely lead to the need for surgical drainage. **Infection** especially in diabetics or immunosuppressed individuals may be severe limb cellulitis and/or systemic and occasionally life-threatening infection. **Injury to the digital nerve(s)** is rare, except when severe scarring is present preoperatively. This may cause **permanent sensory loss**, which the patient should be warned about. Numbness is otherwise rarely an issue. If infection or necrosis occurs, poor cosmesis can result. **Skin necrosis** can occur from tight bandaging, or failure to elevate the limb for the first 48–72 h postoperatively due to poor cooperation. **Recurrence of the tendon sheath constriction** can occur necessitating re-operation, particularly in diabetics, but is unpredictable. Infection of the dominant hand after surgery may significantly impact on function and employment. **Stiffness** can be a significant problem if immobility is prolonged, with **loss of mobility**.

Consent and Risk Reduction

Main Points to Explain

- Discomfort
- Bleeding
- Infection
- Numbness
- Stiffness
- Loss of mobility
- Further surgery

Fig. 4.1 Ganglion of the right thumb dorsal interphalyngeal joint space

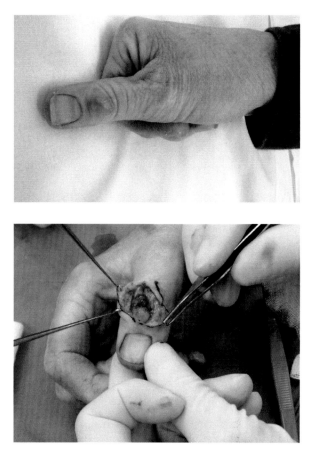

Fig. 4.2 Surgical exposure of the ganglion of the right thumb shown in Fig. 4.1

Surgery for Ganglion Excision

Description

Local anesthesia, axillary arm block, ischemic arm block, or general anesthesia can be used. The aim is to define the origin of the ganglion from the respective joint and excise the ganglion and its neck. Suturing of the fibrous joint capsule and the ganglion neck is often performed using absorbable sutures (Figs. 4.1, 4.2, 4.3, and 4.4).

Anatomical Points

The ganglion is formed by outpouching of the synovial membrane through the degenerated fibrous joint capsule and is filled by clear "jelly" fluid. It is connected to the joint space, or occasionally arises from a tendon sheath, by a narrow "neck."

Fig. 4.3 Ganglion of the
dorsum of the right carpus

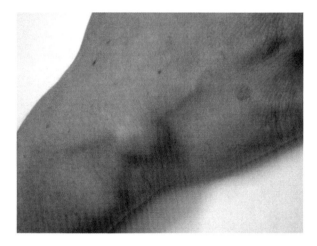

Fig. 4.4 Surgical exposure if
the ganglion shown in
Fig. 4.3, revealing the
gelatinous mass

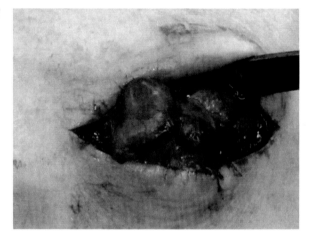

This "neck" may be very narrow and long, such that the ganglion lies well away from the joint site of origin. For this reason careful clinical examination, particularly relating to the mobility and the likely site of origin of the ganglion is very useful for best placing the incision. In general, longitudinal incisions are preferred except perhaps over joint creases and can be designed to permit easy extension if the site of origin of the ganglion might be uncertain. The risk to digital nerves or vessels is determined by the site of the ganglion and incision chosen (Table 4.3).

Perspective

Surgery for ganglion excision is usually very straightforward and complications are few and minor; however, serious complications can be debilitating and occasionally necessitate further surgery. Patients should be aware of the small chance

Table 4.3 Surgery for ganglion excision estimated frequency of complications, risks, and consequences

Complications, risks, and consequences	Estimated frequency
Most significant/serious complications	
Bleeding or hematoma formation	1–5 %
Ganglion recurrence	5–20 %
Inability to correct long-term symptoms (pain)[a]	1–5 %
Numbness and nerve problems	1–5 %
Rare significant/serious problems	
Infection	0.1–1 %
Severe neural injury—digital nerve	0.1–1 %
Necrosis of skin edges/flaps[a]	0.1–1 %
Necessity for skin flaps or grafts	<0.1 %
Dehiscence	<0.1 %
Less serious complications	
Pain/discomfort/tenderness	
Acute (<2 months)	20–50 %
Chronic (>2 months)	1–5 %
Reduced mobility[a]	
Acute (<2 months)	20–50 %
Chronic (>2 months)	0.1–1 %
Bruising	50–80 %
Wound scarring/deformity (poor cosmesis)	1–5 %
Drain tube(s)[a]	<0.1 %

[a]Depends on underlying pathology, state of advancement of disease, surgical technique preferences

of these serious complications. The decision for surgery must be balanced by the risks of the non-operative alternative of observation and conservative management. However, the presence of significant hand discomfort or immobility usually dictates earlier surgical intervention. Postoperative infection may be debilitating especially in diabetic or immunosuppressed individuals and occasionally lead to arm cellulitis and even systemic infections. Excessive pressure from bandages or tight sutures from swelling can lead to local necrosis of the wound edges. Bruising due to slow, concealed postoperative bleeding can cause hand swelling. Recurrence of ganglion formation is not uncommon, particularly at the distal joint level in hand.

Major Complications

Bleeding may rarely be severe, causing a concealed palmar hematoma can rarely lead to the need for surgical drainage. **Infection**, especially in diabetics or immunosuppressed individuals, may lead to severe limb cellulitis and/or systemic and occasionally life-threatening infection. **Injury to the digital nerve(s)** is rare, except when severe scarring is present preoperatively. This may cause permanent sensory loss, which the patient should be warned about. **Numbness** is otherwise rarely an issue. If infection or necrosis occurs, poor cosmesis can result. **Skin**

necrosis can occur from tight bandaging, or failure to elevate the limb for the first 48–72 h postoperatively due to poor cooperation. **Recurrence of the ganglion** can occur necessitating re-operation, but is unpredictable, although not unusual. Development of another separate ganglion may also occur, due to the underlying fibrous joint capsule degenerative problem. Recurrence and new formation of a ganglion may not be able to be deciphered. **Septic arthritis** is rare. Infection of the dominant hand after surgery may significantly impact on function and employment. **Stiffness** can be a significant problem if immobility is prolonged, with **loss of mobility**.

Consent and Risk Reduction

Main Points to Explain

- Discomfort
- Bleeding
- Infection
- Numbness
- Stiffness
- Loss of mobility
- Further surgery

Surgery for Foreign Body Removal

Description

Local anesthesia, regional arm block, ischemic arm block, or general anesthesia can be used. The aim is to define the site and nature of the foreign body in the hand and to locate and remove it with the most minimal injury to surrounding tissues. Imaging, including plain X-ray or ultrasound, may be useful to locate and define the foreign body. Suturing the wound may be performed, or if contaminated, the wound may be left open for delayed primary closure or closure by secondary intention.

Anatomical Points

The nature and location of the foreign body may be able to be determined by the history and investigations (e.g., X-ray or ultrasound) to define the surrounding anatomy. These features will largely determine the operative approach and risks to associated anatomical structures, such as nerves, tendons, joints, or vessels. The risk to digital nerves or vessels is determined by the site of the foreign body, associated

Table 4.4 Surgery for foreign body removal estimated frequency of complications, risks, and consequences

Complications, risks, and consequences	Estimated frequency
Most significant/serious complications	
Bleeding or hematoma formation[a]	1–5 %
Infection[a]	1–5 %
Numbness/altered sensation	1–5 %
Rare significant/serious problems	
Inability to correct long-term symptoms (pain)[a]	0.1–1 %
Sensation of retained material	0.1–1 %
Retention/failure to remove of foreign body[a]	0.1–1 %
Neural injury—digital nerve[a]	0.1–1 %
Necrosis of skin edges/flaps[a]	0.1–1 %
Necessity for skin flaps or grafts[a]	<0.1 %
Dehiscence	<0.1 %
Less serious complications	
Pain/discomfort/tenderness	
Acute (<2 months)	20–50 %
Chronic (>2 months)	1–5 %
Reduced mobility[a]	
Acute (<2 months)	20–50 %
Chronic (>2 months)	0.1–1 %
Bruising	50–80 %
Wound scarring/deformity (poor cosmesis)	1–5 %
Drain tube(s)[a]	<0.1 %

[a]Depends on underlying pathology, type/nature/duration of FB, surgical technique preferences

trauma, and the incision chosen. Image intensification radiology may assist in anatomically locating the foreign body and removal at surgery (Table 4.4).

Perspective

Surgery for foreign body excision is usually very straightforward and complications are few and minor; however, serious complications can be debilitating and occasionally necessitate further surgery. Patients should be aware of the small chance of these serious complications. The decision for surgery must be balanced by the risks of the non-operative alternative of observation and conservative management. However, the presence of significant hand discomfort or immobility usually dictates earlier surgical intervention. Postoperative infection may be debilitating especially in diabetic or immunosuppressed individuals and occasionally lead to arm cellulitis and even systemic infections. Excessive pressure from bandages or tight sutures from swelling can lead to local necrosis of the wound edges. Bruising due to slow, concealed postoperative bleeding can cause hand swelling. Sometimes, the foreign body/material cannot be found, especially if it is small, deep, or radiolucent. The risks of surgical removal should be balanced against careful clinical observation. Certain foreign bodies, for example palm fronds, wood or marine materials, can be particularly irritant and may fragment easily.

Major Complications

Bleeding may rarely be severe, causing a concealed palmar hematoma can rarely lead to the need for surgical drainage. **Infection**, especially in diabetics or immuno-suppressed individuals, may lead to severe limb cellulitis and/or occasionally life-threatening systemic infection. **Injury to the digital nerve(s)** is rare, except when severe scarring is present preoperatively. This may cause permanent sensory loss, which the patient should be warned about. **Numbness** is otherwise rarely an issue. If infection or necrosis occurs, poor cosmesis can result. **Skin necrosis** can occur from tight bandaging, or failure to elevate the limb for the first 48–72 h postopera-tively due to poor cooperation. **Retention of foreign material** or the sensation "that something is still there" can occur necessitating re-operation, but is unusual and unpredictable. Rarely, a tendon or fibrous joint capsule may be breached by the foreign body, leading to difficult access and increased risk of injury with or without surgery. The aim is to minimize the extent of surgery and avoid complications from over-enthusiastic surgical efforts to remove the foreign body. **Septic arthritis** is rare. Infection of the dominant hand after surgery may significantly impact on func-tion and employment. **Stiffness** can be a significant problem if immobility is pro-longed, with **loss of mobility**.

Consent and Risk Reduction

Main Points to Explain

- Discomfort
- Bleeding
- Infection
- Numbness
- Stiffness
- Loss of mobility
- Further surgery

Surgery for Skin Lesion or Dermatofibroma Excision

Description

Local anesthesia, regional arm block, ischemic arm block, or general anesthesia can be used. The aim is to remove the lesion with a small margin of normal tissue with the most minimal injury to surrounding tissues. The wound is usually sutured.

Table 4.5 Surgery for dermatofibroma excision estimated frequency of complications, risks, and consequences

Complications, risks, and consequences	Estimated frequency
Most significant/serious complications	
Bleeding or hematoma formation	1–5 %
Infection	1–5 %
Tumor recurrence[a]	1–5 %
Numbness/altered sensation	1–5 %
Rare significant/serious problems	
Neural injury—digital nerve[a]	0.1–1 %
Necrosis of skin edges/flaps[a]	0.1–1 %
Necessity for skin flaps or grafts	<0.1 %
Dehiscence	<0.1 %
Less serious complications	
Pain/discomfort/tenderness	
Acute (<2 months)	20–50 %
Chronic (>2 months)	0.1–1 %
Reduced mobility[a]	
Acute (<2 months)	20–50 %
Chronic (>2 months)	0.1–1 %
Bruising	50–80 %
Wound scarring/deformity (poor cosmesis)	1–5 %

[a]Depends on underlying pathology, nature/duration of lesion, surgical technique preferences

Anatomical Points

The nature and location of the dermatofibroma/lesion is defined on examination and this will indicate the surrounding anatomy. These features will largely determine the operative approach and risks to associated anatomical structures, such as nerves, tendons, joints, or vessels. The risk to digital nerves or vessels is determined by the site of the lesion and incision chosen (Table 4.5).

Perspective

Surgery for dermatofibroma/lesion excision is usually very straightforward and complications are few and minor; however, serious complications can be debilitating and occasionally necessitate further surgery. Patients should be aware of the small chance of these serious complications. The decision for surgery must be balanced by the risks of the non-operative alternative of observation and conservative management. However, the presence of significant hand discomfort or increasing size usually dictates earlier surgical intervention. Postoperative infection may be debilitating especially in diabetic or immunosuppressed individuals and occasionally lead to arm cellulitis and even systemic infections. Excessive pressure from bandages or tight sutures from swelling can lead to local necrosis of the wound edges. Bruising due to slow, concealed postoperative bleeding can cause hand swelling. The risks of surgical removal should be balanced against careful clinical observation. Dermatofibromas often extend deeper into the subcutaneous fat tissues and require a deeper excision.

Major Complications

Bleeding may rarely be severe, causing a concealed palmar hematoma can rarely lead to the need for surgical drainage. **Infection**, especially in diabetics or immunosuppressed individuals, may lead to severe limb cellulitis and/or occasionally life-threatening systemic infection. **Injury to the digital nerve(s)** is rare, except when the lesion is large or located over/invades a digital nerve. This may cause permanent sensory loss, which the patient should be warned about. **Numbness** is otherwise rarely an issue. If infection or necrosis occurs, poor cosmesis can result. **Skin necrosis** can occur from tight bandaging, or failure to elevate the limb for the first 48–72 h postoperatively due to poor cooperation. **Recurrence** is possible due to the nature of the lesion and the patient should be informed of this risk. **Septic arthritis** is rare. Infection of the dominant hand after surgery may significantly impact on function and employment. **Stiffness** can be a significant problem if immobility is prolonged, with **loss of mobility**.

Consent and Risk Reduction

Main Points to Explain

- Discomfort
- Bleeding
- Infection
- Numbness
- Stiffness
- Loss of mobility
- Further surgery

Surgery for Fingertip Injury (Traumatic)

Description

Local anesthesia, regional arm block, ischemic arm block, or general anesthesia can be used. The aim is to debride and repair the injury using surrounding normal tissue or a skin graft. Restoration of function is the main goal, but sensation and cosmesis are important considerations too. The wound is usually sutured.

Table 4.6 Surgery for fingertip injury (traumatic) estimated frequency of complications, risks, and consequences

Complications, risks, and consequences	Estimated frequency
Most significant/serious complications	
Bleeding or hematoma formation	1–5 %
Infection	1–5 %
Numbness and nerve problems	1–5 %
Shortening of digit[a]	>80 %
Predisposition to arthritis in other joints of the finger	1–5 %
Rare significant/serious problems	
Neural injury—digital nerve[a]	0.1–1 %
Chronic pain[a]	0.1–1 %
Necrosis of skin edges/flaps[a]	0.1–1 %
Dehiscence	<0.1 %
Necessity for skin flaps or grafts	<0.1 %
Less serious complications	
Pain/discomfort/tenderness	
Acute (<2 months)	20–50 %
Chronic (>2 months)	0.1–1 %
Reduced mobility[a]	
Acute (<2 months)	20–50 %
Chronic (>2 months)	0.1–1 %
Bruising	50–80 %
Wound scarring/deformity (poor cosmesis)	1–5 %
Drain tube(s)[a]	<0.1 %

[a]Depends on underlying pathology, nature/duration of lesion, surgical technique preferences

Anatomical Points

The nature and location of fingertip injury is defined on examination and this will indicate the surrounding anatomy and surgical possibilities. These features will largely determine the operative approach and risks to associated anatomical structures, such as nerves, tendons, joints, or vessels. The risk to digital nerves, vessels, pulp, and nail bed is determined by the site of the extent of injury and incisions chosen (Table 4.6).

Perspective

Surgery for fingertip injury is often straightforward and complications are few and minor; however, complex injuries can be challenging and serious complications can be debilitating and occasionally necessitate further surgery. Patients should be aware of the small chance of these serious complications. The decision for surgery must be balanced, where possible, by possible risks of non-operative approaches and more conservative management. However, the presence of significant hand discomfort, deformity, or infection risk usually dictates earlier surgical intervention. Postoperative infection may be debilitating especially in diabetic or immunosuppressed individuals and occasionally lead to arm cellulitis and even systemic infections. Compound bone or joint injury increases the risk of osteomyelitis or septic arthritis. Excessive pressure from bandages or tight sutures from swelling can lead to local necrosis of the wound edges. Bruising due to slow, concealed postoperative bleeding can cause hand swelling. The risks of surgical removal should be balanced against careful clinical nonintervention.

Major Complications

Bleeding may rarely be severe, causing a concealed palmar hematoma can rarely lead to the need for surgical drainage. **Infection** especially in diabetics or immunosuppressed individuals may cause severe limb cellulitis and/or occasionally life-threatening systemic infection. **Injury to the digital nerve(s)** is rare, except when the injury is large or involves a digital nerve. This may cause permanent sensory loss, which the patient should be warned about. **Numbness** is otherwise rarely an issue. If infection or necrosis occurs, poor cosmesis can result. **Skin necrosis** can occur from tight bandaging, or failure to elevate the limb for the first 48–72 h postoperatively due to poor cooperation. **Chronic pain**, discharging infection, poor cosmesis, shortening of the digit(s), and loss of function are serious problems and the patient should be informed of these risks, ideally before surgery. **Septic arthritis** is rare. Infection of the dominant hand after surgery may significantly impact on function and employment. **Stiffness** can be a significant problem if immobility is prolonged, with **loss of mobility**.

Consent and Risk Reduction

Main Points to Explain

- Discomfort
- Bleeding
- Infection
- Numbness
- Stiffness
- Loss of mobility
- Further surgery

Surgery for Dupuytren's (Contracture): Palmar Fasciectomy

Description

Local anesthesia, regional arm block, ischemic arm block, or general anesthesia can be used. The aim is to release and excise the contracted palmar fascia tissue using surrounding normal tissue or a skin graft. Restoration of hand function is the goal. The wound is usually sutured.

Anatomical Points

Dupuytren's contracture is due to a thickening of the tissue between the skin and palmar aponeurosis and classically involves both structures. The palmar aspect proximal to the ring finger is commonly affected, typically producing flexion contracture of the ring finger. The nature and location of the Dupuytren's contracture is defined on examination and this will indicate the surrounding anatomy and surgical possibilities. These features will largely determine the operative approach and risks to associated anatomical structures, such as nerves, tendons, joints, or vessels. The risk to digital nerves, vessels, tendons, and skin is determined by the site of the extent of the contracture and incisions chosen (Table 4.7).

Perspective

Surgery for Dupuytren's contracture is usually straightforward and complications are few and minor; however, serious complications can be debilitating and occasionally necessitate further surgery. Patients should be aware of the small chance of these serious complications. The contracture can be severe and complex necessitating more complex surgery with increased risks. The decision for surgery must be balanced by the risks of the non-operative alternative of observation and conservative management. However, the presence of significant hand discomfort or immobility usually dictates earlier surgical intervention. Postoperative infection may be debilitating especially in diabetic or immunosuppressed individuals and occasionally lead to arm cellulitis and even systemic infections. Excessive pressure from bandages or tight sutures from swelling can lead to local necrosis of the wound edges. Bruising due to slow, concealed postoperative bleeding can cause hand swelling.

Table 4.7 Surgery for Dupuytren's palmar fasciectomy (Dupuytren's contracture) estimated frequency of complications, risks, and consequences

Complications, risks, and consequences	Estimated frequency
Most significant/serious complications	
Bleeding or hematoma formation	1–5 %
Infection	1–5 %
Reformation of the Dupuytren's contracture[a,b]	5–10 %
Numbness/altered sensation[a,b]	5–10 %
Failure to fully relieve PIP contracture[a,b]	5–10 %
Rare significant/serious problems	
Inability to correct long-term symptoms (weakness; anesthesia, or paresthesia)	0.1–1 %
Neural injury—digital nerve(s)[a]	0.1–1 %
Necrosis of skin edges/flaps/palmar skin[a]	0.1–1 %
Necessity for skin flaps or grafts[a]	<0.1 %
Dehiscence	<0.1 %
Less serious complications	
Pain/discomfort/tenderness	
Acute (<2 months)	20–50 %
Chronic (>2 months)	0.1–1 %
Reduced mobility[a]	
Acute (<2 months)	20–50 %
Chronic (>2 months)	0.1–1 %
Bruising	50–80 %
Wound scarring/deformity (poor cosmesis)	1–5 %
Drain tube(s)[a]	<0.1 %

[a]Depends on underlying pathology, extent/nature/duration of lesion, age of the patient at surgery, surgical technique preferences
[b]The extent of all of these complications is often determined by the age of the patient and severity of the contracture at surgery

Major Complications

Bleeding may rarely be severe, causing a concealed palmar hematoma can rarely lead to the need for surgical drainage. **Infection**, especially in diabetics or immuno-suppressed individuals, may lead to severe limb cellulitis and/or systemic and occasionally life-threatening. **Injury to the digital nerve(s)** is possible, especially when severe scarring is present preoperatively, or from recurrent disease. This may cause permanent sensory loss, which the patient should be warned about. **Numbness** is otherwise rarely an issue. If infection or necrosis occurs, poor cosmesis can result. **Skin necrosis** can occur from tight bandaging, or failure to elevate the limb for the first 48–72 h postoperatively due to poor cooperation. This can occasionally be serious and involve large areas of the palmar skin, and rarely even require **skin grafting**. **Recurrence** of the contracture can occur necessitating re-operation, which is not unusual and is unpredictable. Infection of the dominant hand after surgery may significantly impact on function and employment. **Stiffness** can be a significant problem if immobility is prolonged, with **loss of mobility**.

Consent and Risk Reduction

Main Points to Explain

- Discomfort
- Bleeding
- Infection
- Numbness
- Stiffness
- Loss of mobility
- Further surgery

Further Reading, References, and Resources

Clemente CD. Anatomy – a regional atlas of the human body. 4th ed. Baltimore: Williams and Wilkins; 1997.

Jamieson GG. The anatomy of general surgical operations. 2nd ed. Edinburgh: Churchill Livingston; 2006.

Thorne CH, Bartlett SP, Beasley RW, Aston SJ. Grabb's plastic surgery. 6th ed. Philadelphia: Lippincott Williams and Wilkins; 2006. ISBN 978-0781746984.

Wolfe SW, Pederson WC, Hotchkiss RN, Kozin SH. Green's operative hand surgery. 6th ed. Philadelphia: Churchill Livingstone; 2011 (Online and Print). ISBN 978-1416052791.

Chapter 5
Foot Surgery

Brendon J. Coventry and Peter Stavrou

General Perspective and Overview

The relative risks and complications increase proportionately according to the type of foot problem, site and size of lesion/problem, extent of procedure performed, technique, imaging guidance (if needed), and the lesion size. Complications overall are more likely more distally in the lower limb because of progressively poorer vascularity. Any further compromise to vascular supply, such as age, diabetes, peripheral vascular disease, lymphedema, or injury, usually will reduce healing capacity, or the effects of peripheral neuropathy should be considered. Large excisions in highly vascular tissues carry higher risk of bleeding than for less vascular structures. Similarly, the risk of numbness and nerve problems is relatively higher for larger and deeper lesion excisions performed closer to neural structures (e.g., digital nerves). With regard to scarring, it needs to be explained to the patient that some scarring is usual, but if the lesion is not removed with surgery, the consequence may be far more of a problem (depending on the pathology). Flaps and grafts require an explanation of the possibility of partial or total failure, and the need for dressings and/or further surgery. The risks of graft donor site complications also need to be considered, in addition to the wound site complications. Failure of the patient to maintain sufficient elevation of the lower limb following surgery will typically lead to congestion due to dependency and consequent increased risk of many complications.

Possible reduction in the risk of misunderstandings over complications or consequences from foot surgery might be achieved by:
- Good explanation of the risks, aims, benefits, and limitations of the procedure
- Useful planning considering the anatomy, approach, alternatives, and method

B.J. Coventry, BMBS, PhD, FRACS, FACS, FRSM (✉) • P. Stavrou, MBBS, FRACS, FA, Ortho A
Discipline of Surgery, Royal Adelaide Hospital, University of Adelaide,
L5 Eleanor Harrald Building, North Terrace, 5000 Adelaide, SA, Australia
e-mail: brendon.coventry@adelaide.edu.au

B.J. Coventry (ed.), *Peripheral, Head and Neck Surgery*,
Surgery: Complications, Risks and Consequences,
DOI 10.1007/978-1-4471-5415-0_5, © Springer-Verlag London 2014

- Avoiding/protecting likely associated vessels and nerves
- Appropriate patient selection
- Adequate clinical follow-up
- Explanation of the expected range of functional outcomes of the procedure to manage patient expectations.

With these factors and facts in mind, the information given in this chapter must be appropriately and discernibly interpreted and used.

IMPORTANT NOTE: It should be emphasized that the risks and frequencies that are given here *represent derived figures*. These *figures are best estimates of relative frequencies across most institutions*, not merely the highest-performing ones, and as such are often representative of a number of studies, which include different patients with differing comorbidities and different surgeons. In addition, the risks of complications in lower or higher risk patients may lie outside these estimated ranges, and individual clinical judgement is required as to the expected risks communicated to the patient, staff, or for other purposes. The range of risks is also derived from experience and the literature; while risks outside this range may exist, certain risks may be reduced or absent due to variations of procedures or surgical approaches. It is recognized that different patients, practitioners, institutions, regions, and countries may vary in their requirements and recommendations.

For diagnostic needle biopsies of lesions (Chap. 2) or excision of skin lesions (Chap. 3), or other biopsies used to obtain diagnosis, please refer to the relevant volume and chapter.

Surgery for Wedge Resection of Ingrowing Toenail

Description

Local anesthesia, usually using regional ring blockade, or general anesthesia may be used. The aim is to excise the lateral edge of the ingrowing toenail including the underlying nail bed by removing a tissue wedge. The excision must include the germinal matrix proximal to the nail fold.

Anatomical Points

The nail excessively folds around the lateral edge of the nail bed and ingrows into the lateral pulp of the toe. The nail bed extends proximally below the skin at the nail fold and excision must include all of the nail, nail bed and the germinal matrix more proximal still to the nail to prevent regrowth of the nail. The excised tissue should extend almost to the distal interphalangeal metatarsal joint, but not breach the joint capsule. The germinal matrix is often adherent to the distal phalanx and requires curettage to adequately remove the germinal tissue from which the nail can regrow. The length of the distal phalanx itself and the proximity of the germinal matrix to the distal interphalangeal joint can vary between individuals. Note that anatomically, the hallux has only one interphalangeal joint (Table 5.1).

Perspective

Surgery for excision of ingrowing toenail is usually very straightforward and complications are few and minor; however, serious complications can be debilitating and necessitate further surgery. Patients should be aware of the small chance of

Table 5.1 Surgery for wedge resection of ingrown toenail estimated frequency of complications, risks, and consequences

Complications, risks, and consequences	Estimated frequency
Most significant/serious complications	
Bleeding or hematoma formation	5–20 %
Infection[a]	1–5 %
Aberrant nail regrowth[a]	5–20 %
Severe deformity of the nail[a]	1–5 %
Recurrence of ingrowing toenail[a]	1–5 %
Rare significant/serious problems	
Osteomyelitis (very rare)	<0.1 %
Septic arthritis (very rare)	<0.1 %
Skin flaps or grafts	<0.1 %
Less serious complications	
Pain/discomfort/tenderness	
Acute (<2 months)	50–80 %
Chronic (>2 months)	0.1–1 %
Reduced mobility[a]	
Acute (<2 months)	20–50 %
Chronic (>2 months)	0.1–1 %
Numbness/altered sensation	1–5 %
Bruising	>80 %
Scarring	1–5 %
Dimpling/deformity of the skin	>80 %
Granulation tissue formation	1–5 %
Wound dehiscence[a]	<0.1 %

[a]Depends on underlying pathology, state of advancement of disease, surgical technique

these serious complications. The decision for surgery must be balanced by the non-operative alternative of antibiotic therapy and conservative management. Recurrent infection may be debilitating and in some patients, such as diabetics or immunosuppressed individuals can lead to gait disturbances, lower limb cellulitis, systemic infections, or very rarely osteomyelitis and toe necrosis. The ingrowing toenail may be subject to recurrent infections and it is prudent to avoid surgery in the acute infected state. Surgery should be postponed during active infection and treated with antibiotics until further clinical review prior to undertaking surgery. Recurrence of the ingrowing toenail can occur at the same site or involve the other side of the toenail. Should the toenail ingrown on both borders, Zadik's procedure should be considered because bilateral wedge resections may lead to a narrow nail with obvious cosmetic issues. Bilateral ingrowing toenails are most commonly seen in teenage boys.

Major Complications

Bleeding may be severe and rarely leads to the need for surgical drainage. **Infection** especially in diabetics or immunosuppressed individuals may be systemic and occasionally even life-threatening. **Bone or joint infections** are very rare, but are potentially very serious complications that are chronic and debilitating, necessitating prolonged antibiotic therapy and sometimes further surgery. **Recurrence** of the ingrowing toenail is not uncommon depending on the technique. The nail remnant is often quite troublesome for the patient as it can protrude from the nail bed at an odd angle, catching on socks. This will often necessitate revision surgery. **Numbness** is rarely an issue. **Gait difficulties** are a consequence of infection or **joint stiffness/fusion**, but may arise without surgery. **Cosmesis can be poor**; however, the preoperative ingrowing toenail can also be unsightly in appearance. It is useful to advise the patient about the potential for deformity of the remaining nail.

Consent and Risk Reduction

Main Points to Explain

- Recurrence
- Discomfort
- Bleeding
- Infection
- Poor cosmesis
- Loss of mobility
- Further surgery

Surgery for Ingrowing Toenail Nail bed Ablation (Zadik's Procedure)

Description

Local anesthesia, usually using regional ring blockade or general anesthesia may be used. The aim is to excise the *entire* nail and proximal part of the nail bed including the ingrowing toenail to prevent regrowth and recurrence. The excision must include the germinal matrix proximal to the nail fold.

Anatomical Variance

The nail folds around the lateral edge of the nail bed and ingrows into the lateral pulp of the toe. The nail bed extends below the skin proximally at the nail fold and excision must include all of the nail, proximal nail bed and the germinal matrix more proximal still to the nail to prevent regrowth of the nail. The excised tissue should extend almost to the distal metatarsal joint, but not breach the joint capsule. The germinal matrix is often adherent to the distal phalanx and requires curettage to adequately remove the germinal tissue from which the nail can regrow. The length of the distal phalanx itself and the proximity of the germinal matrix to the distal interphalangeal joint varies between individuals (Table 5.2).

Perspective

Even radical nail surgery for excision of ingrowing toenail is usually very straightforward and complications are few and minor; however, serious complications can be debilitating and necessitate further surgery. Patients should be aware of the small chance of these serious complications. The decision for surgery must be balanced by the nonoperative alternative of antibiotic therapy and conservative management. Recurrent infection may be debilitating and in some patients, such as diabetics or immunosuppressed individuals can lead to gait disturbances, lower limb cellulitis, systemic infections, or very rarely osetomyelitis and toe necrosis. Recurrence of the nail and ingrowing nail can occur, but is very rare when the full nail bed has been removed properly.

Major Complications

Bleeding may be severe and rarely lead to the need for surgical drainage. **Infection** especially in diabetics or immunosuppressed individuals may be systemic and occasionally even life-threatening. **Bone or joint infections** are very rare, but are

Table 5.2 Surgery for ingrown toenail nail bed ablation (Zadik's procedure) estimated frequency of complications, risks, and consequences

Complications, risks, and consequences	Estimated frequency
Most significant/serious complications	
Bleeding or hematoma formation	5–20 %
Infection[a]	1–5 %
Total loss of nail (the aim/consequence)[a]	100 %
Reduced protection of toe (increased risk of injury)[a]	>8v0 %
Rare significant/serious problems	
Minor nail regrowth (recurrence)[a]	0.1–1 %
Osteomyelitis (very rare)	<0.1 %
Septic arthritis (very rare)	<0.1 %
Skin flaps or grafts	<0.1 %
Wound dehiscence	<0.1 %
Less serious complications	
Pain/discomfort/tenderness	
Acute (<2 months)	50–80 %
Chronic (>2 months)	0.1–1 %
Reduced mobility[a]	
Acute (<2 months)	20–50 %
Chronic (>2 months)	0.1–1 %
Bruising	>80 %
Scarring	1–5 %
Dimpling/deformity of the skin[a]	>80 %
Numbness/altered sensation	1–5 %
Granulation tissue formation	1–5 %

[a]Depends on underlying pathology, state of advancement of disease, surgical technique

potentially very serious complications that are chronic and debilitating, necessitating prolonged antibiotic therapy and sometimes further surgery. **Recurrence** of the nail is very rare, but can be quite troublesome as the nail remnant protrudes from the remainder of the nail at an odd angle and often catches on socks. **Numbness** is rarely an issue. **Gait difficulties** are a consequence of infection or joint stiffness/fusion, but may arise without surgery. **Cosmesis can be poor**; the nail is replaced by thickened skin, which may have a less noticeable appearance than the premorbid nail. However, the preoperative ingrowing toenail can also be unsightly in appearance. The **permanent loss of the toenail** increases the risk of **injury to the toe** and may cause considerable discomfort with certain footwear which can be a very significant problem for the patient.

Consent and Risk Reduction

Main Points to Explain

- Discomfort
- Nail remnant/recurrence

- Bleeding
- Infection
- Loss of mobility
- Further surgery

Surgery for Foreign Body Removal

Description

Local anesthesia, regional foot block, peripheral nerve blocks, ischemic leg block, or general anesthesia can be used. The aim is to define the site and nature of the foreign body in the foot and to locate and remove it with the most minimal injury to surrounding tissues. Suturing the wound may be performed, or if contaminated the wound may be left open. Image intensification may be used if the foreign material is radiopaque, or ultrasound (pre- or intra-operative) may be helpful. If a tourniquet is used for the procedure, it should be released prior to wound closure to ensure good hemostasis (Fig. 5.1).

Anatomical Variance

The nature and location of the foreign body may be able to be determined by the history and investigations (e.g., X-ray or ultrasound) to define the surrounding anatomy. These features will largely determine the operative approach and risks to associated anatomical structures, such as nerves, tendons, joints, or vessels. The risk to digital nerves or vessels is determined by the site of the foreign body and incision chosen. Image intensification radiology may assist significantly in anatomically locating the foreign body visible on X-ray and removal at surgery. Ultrasound may be useful for defining non-radiopaque foreign material. Avoid if possible incisions

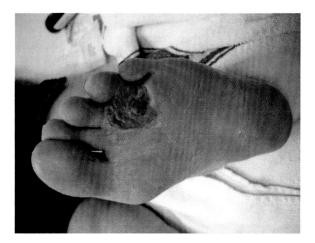

Fig. 5.1 Wound breakdown from a skin graft to the sole of the foot after (delayed) foreign body removal and subsequent wound infection

Table 5.3 Surgery for foreign body removal estimated frequency of complications, risks, and consequences

Complications, risks, and consequences	Estimated frequency
Most significant/serious complications	
Bleeding or hematoma formation[a]	1–5 %
Infection[a]	1–5 %
Rare significant/serious problems	
Neural injury—digital nerve[a]	0.1–1 %
Inability to correct long-term symptoms (pain)[a]	0.1–1 %
Sensation of retained material[a]	0.1–1 %
Retention/failure to remove of foreign body[a]	0.1–1 %
Necrosis of skin edges/flaps[a]	0.1–1 %
Necessity for skin flaps or grafts[a]	<0.1 %
Dehiscence	<0.1 %
Less serious complications	
Pain/discomfort/tenderness	
Acute (<2 months)	0.1–1 %
Chronic (>2 months)	0.1–1 %
Reduced mobility[a]	
Acute (<2 months)	0.1–1 %
Chronic (>2 months)	0.1–1 %
Bruising	50–80 %
Numbness/altered sensation	1–5 %
Wound scarring/deformity (poor cosmesis)	1–5 %
Drain tube(s)[a]	<0.1 %

[a]Depends on underlying pathology, nature/duration of FB, surgical technique preferences

on the weight-bearing surface of the foot. Be familiar with the anatomy of the medial and lateral plantar nerves, as altered sensation in the weight-bearing aspect of the foot can cause significant morbidity (Table 5.3).

Perspective

Surgery for foreign body excision can be very straightforward and complications are few and minor; however, serious complications can be debilitating and occasionally necessitate further surgery. Patients should be aware of the small chance of these serious complications. The decision for surgery must be balanced by the non-operative alternative of observation and conservative management. However, the presence of significant foot discomfort or immobility usually dictates earlier surgical intervention. Postoperative infection may be debilitating especially in diabetic or immunosuppressed individuals and occasionally lead to foot cellulitis and even systemic infections. Excessive pressure from bandages or tight sutures from swelling can lead to local necrosis of the wound edges. Bruising due to slow, concealed postoperative bleeding can cause foot swelling. Image intensification is often very useful in locating the foreign body, especially metal or glass. Sometimes, the foreign body/material cannot be found, especially if it is small, deep, or radiolucent. Removal of only part of the material can occur, especially if the material fragments easily or is in multiple parts. Certain foreign bodies, for example palm fronds, wood or marine materials, can be particularly irritant and may fragment easily. The risks of surgical removal should be balanced against the risks of careful clinical observation. Organic materials such as palm fronds, wood or marine materials are usually radiolucent, these are best identified with ultrasound preoperatively. In the presence of ongoing problems postoperatively ultrasound should be undertaken to exclude any retained foreign body. Glass and metal are radiopaque and image intensification can be utilized intra-operatively. It should be noted that glass is almost impossible to see in a bloodsoaked wound and should be felt with a forceps rather than the surgeon's finger. If there is any doubt, screening with image intensification should be undertaken during and prior to wound closure to avoid any retained fragments of foreign body.

Major Complications

Bleeding is rarely severe, and a concealed hematoma can rarely lead to the need for surgical drainage. **Infection** especially in diabetics or immunosuppressed individuals may cause severe limb cellulitis and/or occasionally life-threatening systemic infection. **Injury to the digital nerve(s)** is rare, except when severe scarring is present preoperatively. This may cause permanent sensory loss, which the patient should be warned about. **Numbness** is otherwise rarely an issue. If infection or necrosis occurs, poor cosmesis can result. Tissue necrosis can occur from tight bandaging, or failure to elevate the limb for the first 48–72 h postoperatively due to poor cooperation. **Retention of foreign material** or the sensation "that something is still there" can occur necessitating re-operation, but is unusual and unpredictable. Rarely, a tendon or fibrous joint capsule may be breached by the foreign body leading to difficult access and increased risk of injury with or without surgery. The aim is to minimize the extent of surgery and avoid complications from over-enthusiastic surgical efforts to remove the foreign body. Scar tenderness, scars over the weight-bearing aspect of the foot can cause long-term discomfort and should be avoided if possible.

Consent and Risk Reduction

Main Points to Explain

- Discomfort
- Bleeding
- Infection
- Loss of mobility

- Retention of foreign body
- Further surgery

Surgery for Ganglion Excision

Description

Local anesthesia, foot block, ischemic leg block, or general anesthesia can be used. The aim is to define the origin of the ganglion from the respective joint and excise the ganglion at its origin. Suturing of the fibrous joint capsule and the ganglion neck is often performed using absorbable sutures.

Anatomical Variance

The ganglion is connected to the joint space, or occasionally arises from a tendon sheath, by a "neck." This "neck" may be narrowed and can be very long, such that the ganglion lies away from the site of origin. For this reason careful clinical examination, particularly relating to the mobility and likely site of origin of the ganglion is very useful in best placing the incision. Ultrasound can be used to identify the origin of the ganglion. The narrow neck of the ganglion can act as a valve; to eliminate this effect after excision of the ganglion the capsular defect can either be sutured or expanded so as not to allow a narrow neck to form. In general, longitudinal incisions are preferred except perhaps over joint creases and can be designed to permit easy extension if the site of origin of the ganglion might be uncertain. The risk to digital nerves or vessels is determined by the site of the ganglion and incision chosen (Table 5.4).

Perspective

Surgery for ganglion excision is usually very straightforward and complications are few and minor; however, serious complications can be debilitating and occasionally necessitate further surgery. Patients should be aware of the small chance of these serious complications. The decision for surgery must be balanced by the nonoperative alternative of observation and conservative management. However, the presence of significant foot discomfort or immobility usually dictates earlier surgical intervention. Postoperative infection may be debilitating especially in diabetic or immunosuppressed individuals and occasionally lead to foot cellulitis and even systemic infections. Excessive pressure from bandages or tight sutures from

Table 5.4 Surgery for ganglion excision estimated frequency of complications, risks, and consequences

Complications, risks, and consequences	Estimated frequency
Most significant/serious complications	
Bleeding or hematoma formation	1–5 %
Ganglion recurrence	1–5 %
Inability to correct long-term symptoms (pain)[a]	1–5 %
Numbness/altered sensation	1–5 %
Rare significant/serious problems	
Infection	0.1–1 %
Severe neural injury—digital nerve	0.1–1 %
Necrosis of skin edges/flaps[a]	0.1–1 %
Necessity for skin flaps or grafts[a]	<0.1 %
Dehiscence	<0.1 %
Less serious complications	
Pain/discomfort/tenderness	
Acute (<2 months)	20–50 %
Chronic (>2 months)	0.1–1 %
Reduced mobility[a]	
Acute (<2 months)	20–50 %
Chronic (>2 months)	0.1–1 %
Bruising	50–80 %
Wound scarring/deformity (poor cosmesis)	1–5 %

[a]Depends on underlying pathology, state of advancement of disease, surgical technique preferences

swelling can lead to local necrosis of the wound edges. Bruising due to slow, concealed postoperative bleeding can cause foot swelling.

Major Complications

Bleeding may rarely be severe, causing a concealed hematoma can rarely lead to the need for surgical drainage. **Infection** especially in diabetics or immunosuppressed individuals may be severe limb cellulitis and/or systemic and occasionally life-threatening. **Injury to the digital nerve(s)** is rare, except when severe scarring is present preoperatively. This may cause permanent sensory loss, which the patient should be warned about. **Numbness** is otherwise rarely an issue. If infection or necrosis occurs, poor cosmesis can result. Tissue necrosis can occur from tight bandaging, or failure to elevate the limb for the first 48–72 h postoperatively due to poor cooperation. **Reformation or recurrence of the ganglion** can occur necessitating re-operation, but is not unusual and unpredictable. Development of another separate ganglion may also occur, due to the underlying fibrous joint capsule degenerative problem. Recurrence and new formation of a ganglion may be unable to be deciphered. Foot infection may very significantly impede mobility.

Consent and Risk Reduction

Main Points to Explain

- Recurrence of ganglion
- Discomfort
- Bleeding
- Infection
- Loss of mobility
- Further surgery

Surgery for Hammertoe Correction

Description

Local anesthesia, regional foot block, ischemic leg block, or general anesthesia can be used. The aim is to excise the proximal/middle phalanx in order to straighten the toe. This usually alleviates the crossing over of adjacent toes. Suturing of the wound is performed. The surgical technique is dependent upon the pathology encountered in the patient. Flexible/correctable deformities can often be treated with soft tissue procedures such as flexor or extensor tenotomy. Fixed deformity will require bony correction. Deformity at MTP joint may require soft tissue or bony surgery at this level.

Anatomical Variance

The nature and location of the hammertoe is determined by the history and investigations (e.g., X-ray) to define the anatomy. These features will largely determine the operative approach and risks to associated anatomical structures, such as nerves, tendons, joints, or vessels. The risk to digital nerves or vessels is determined by the severity of the hammertoe and incision chosen. Radiology may assist in anatomically designing the surgery (Table 5.5).

Perspective

Surgery for hammertoe correction is usually very straightforward and complications are few and minor; however, serious complications can be debilitating and occasionally necessitate further surgery. Patients should be aware of the small

Table 5.5 Surgery for hammertoe correction estimated frequency of complications, risks, and consequences

Complications, risks, and consequences	Estimated frequency
Most significant/serious complications	
Bleeding or hematoma formation[a]	1–5 %
Infection[a]	1–5 %
Recurrence/reformation of the hammertoe deformity[a]	1–5 %
Numbness/altered sensation	1–5 %
Rare significant/serious problems	
Inability to correct long-term symptoms (pain)[a]	0.1–1 %
Neural injury—digital nerve[a]	0.1–1 %
Necrosis of skin edges/flaps[a]	0.1–1 %
Long-term mobility problems[a]	0.1–1 %
Necessity for skin flaps or grafts[a]	<0.1 %
Dehiscence	<0.1 %
Vascular injury leading to toe amputation	<0.1 %
Less serious complications	
Pain/discomfort/tenderness	
Acute (<2 months)	20–50 %
Chronic (>2 months)	0.1–1 %
Reduced mobility[a]	
Acute (<2 months)	5–20 %
Chronic (>2 months)	0.1–1 %
Bruising	>80 %
Wound scarring/deformity (poor cosmesis)	5–20 %

[a]Depends on underlying pathology, nature/duration, surgical technique preferences

chance of these serious complications. The decision for surgery must be balanced by the non-operative alternative of observation and conservative management. However, the presence of significant foot discomfort or immobility usually dictates earlier surgical intervention. Postoperative infection may be debilitating especially in diabetic or immunosuppressed individuals and occasionally lead to foot cellulitis and even systemic infections. Excessive pressure from bandages or tight sutures from swelling can lead to local necrosis of the wound edges. Bruising due to slow, concealed postoperative bleeding can cause foot swelling. The risks of surgical correction should be balanced against clinical observation.

Major Complications

Bleeding may rarely be severe, causing a concealed hematoma can rarely lead to the need for surgical drainage. **Infection** especially in diabetics or immunosuppressed individuals may cause severe limb cellulitis and/or occasionally life-threatening systemic infection. **Injury to the digital nerve(s)** is rare, except when severe scarring is present preoperatively. This may cause permanent sensory loss, which the patient should be warned about. **Numbness** is otherwise rarely an issue. If infection or necrosis occurs, **poor cosmesis** can result. **Tissue necrosis** can occur from tight bandaging, or failure to elevate the limb for the first 48–72 h postoperatively due to poor cooperation. **Osteomyelitis** is very rare, but if it occurs can be severely debilitating and require chronic antibiotic therapy and occasionally further surgery. Injury to both digital arteries will lead to necrosis of the toe requiring amputation, this is a rare occurrence. Previous toe or forefoot surgery increases the risk of neurovascular injury, the patient should be warned of this. If there are concerns a digital Allen test or duplex ultrasound can be performed to ensure both digital arteries are patent.

Consent and Risk Reduction

Main Points to Explain

- Discomfort
- Recurrent deformity
- Loss of mobility
- Bleeding
- Infection
- Further surgery

Further Reading, References, and Resources

Clemente CD. Anatomy – a regional atlas of the human body. 4th ed. Baltimore: Williams and Wilkins; 1997.
Jamieson GG. The anatomy of general surgical operations. 2nd ed. Edinburgh: Churchill Livingston; 2006.

Chapter 6
Hernia Surgery

A. Gerson Greenburg and Brendon J. Coventry

General Perspective and Overview

The relative risks and complications increase proportionately according to the site of the hernia, extent of procedure performed, technique, the complexity of the hernia, the hernia size, and importantly individual patient factors. Large herniae surgery carries higher risks of bleeding and infection than smaller ones, in general terms. Similarly, risk is relatively higher for recurrent and complex hernias, and for those closer to neural structures (e.g., ilioinguinal or femoral nerve).

With regard to inguinal hernia, the trans-abdominal pre-peritoneal (TAPP) or total extraperitoneal (TEP) laparoscopic "repair" approaches are to the posterior abdominal wall of the inguinal canal, whereas open hernia repairs are usually repairs to the anterior abdominal wall; however, there are some proponents of the pre-peritoneal open approach also. Therefore, complications with each approach are often related to anatomy that is dissected and associated technical issues. In general, the complications are similar in type. Knowledge of the anatomy and the variations commonly seen is helpful in minimizing nerve and vessel injury, especially to the retroperitoneal structures in the TEP and the intra-abdominal structures in the TAPP approach. Vascular and bowel injury are more likely with these repairs and there is an increased, yet still low level of risk for bladder injury. It must be noted that the intra-abdominal complications associated with laparoscopic access add a

A.G. Greenburg, MD, PhD
Clinical Quality Management, Department of General Surgery,
The Miriam Hospital, Brown University Medical School, Providence, RI, USA

B.J. Coventry, BMBS, PhD, FRACS, FACS, FRSM (✉)
Discipline of Surgery, Royal Adelaide Hospital, University of Adelaide,
L5 Eleanor Harrald Building, North Terrace, 5000 Adelaide, SA, Australia
e-mail: brendon.coventry@adelaide.edu.au

B.J. Coventry (ed.), *Peripheral, Head and Neck Surgery*,
Surgery: Complications, Risks and Consequences,
DOI 10.1007/978-1-4471-5415-0_6, © Springer-Verlag London 2014

new dimension of complications not usually associated with hernia repair. These are more frequent in the TAPP approach it being trans-peritoneal access thus putting the intra-abdominal contents at increased risk for injury. It must be stated that both of the laparoscopic repairs are rooted in information gleaned from the development of the open pre-peritoneal repair of groin hernia. It is fairly appreciated that the complication rates between the two laparoscopic repairs are quite similar. Recurrence rates are low, but still definable for each and may relate to the "learning curve" of experience, as would any new procedure. Surgeons argue the benefits of one approach over the other, but there is really little data to demonstrate differences in terms of the observed or reported complications. Other surgeons will argue that the use of general anesthesia for this approach adds to the complication rates but that is less of a consideration in the current era. Bowel and bladder injury, more common with these approaches, may reflect the surgeon's experience and theoretically should be minimized with more experience. However, there is an intrinsic complication rate associated with the laparoscopic approach that may never be eliminated, perhaps at best minimized by experience.

Another consideration concerning hernia repair generally is the type and use of foreign materials, typically synthetic in origin, for suturing or mesh support. These materials are constantly evolving and do not always have identical properties to each other. This point needs to be borne in mind when evaluating the literature regarding the comparison of different techniques or studies. When these considerations are combined with technical operative factors and individual patient factors, evaluation needs to be carefully performed. One of the main problems is lack of uniformity between (or even within) studies, such that very large numbers of cases require inclusion in each arm of the study groups to ensure sufficient power exists to detect even small differences in outcomes for the various forms of hernia repair. The other issue is the requirement for sufficiently long-term follow-up of the order of 10–20 years, in order to accurately determine outcomes such as hernia recurrence rates.

Possible reduction in the risk of misunderstandings over complications or consequences from hernia surgery might be achieved by:

- Good explanation of the risks, aims, benefits, and limitations of the procedure(s)
- Careful planning considering the anatomy, approach, alternatives, and method
- Avoiding likely associated vessels and nerves
- Adequate clinical follow-up

With these factors and facts in mind, the information given in this chapter must be appropriately and discernibly interpreted and used.

IMPORTANT NOTE: It should be emphasized that the risks and frequencies that are given here *represent derived figures*. These *figures are best estimates of relative frequencies across most institutions*, not merely the highest-performing ones, and as such are often representative of a number of studies, which include different patients with differing comorbidities and different surgeons. In addition, the risks of complications in lower or higher risk patients may lie outside these estimated ranges, and individual clinical judgement is required as to the expected risks communicated to the patient, staff, or for other purposes. The range of risks is also derived from experience and the literature; while risks outside this range may exist, certain risks may be reduced or absent due to variations of procedures or surgical approaches. It is recognized that different patients, practitioners, institutions, regions, and countries may vary in their requirements and recommendations.

For risks and complications associated with full laparotomy, please see volume 4 or the relevant chapter.

Surgery for Epigastric Hernia

Description

General anesthesia is usually used; however, local infiltration can be used in selected cases, with or without systemic neuroleptic agents. The aim of the procedure is to define the hernia sac, excise it, and repair the defect. Either a longitudinal midline or transverse skin incision is used. Epigastric hernia is a relatively common surgical problem. It typically occurs in the midline region between the umbilicus and xyphoid as a bulge, emphasized by coughing. It is a defect in the linea alba allowing abdominal contents to protrude, sometimes containing peritoneum. Occasionally, multiple defects are present. The contents are often pre-peritoneal fat from the falciform ligament, and occasionally omentum and less commonly bowel within a peritoneal sac. It is observed in all ages and both genders almost equally. In obese patients, the diagnosis may be especially difficult. Elective repair is indicated in symptomatic patients; incarceration and bowel obstruction require emergency intervention. The sac is defined and excised at the edge of the linea defect to expose the contents before reduction. A midline longitudinal incision above and/or below the linea alba defect is usual to extend the hernial opening if better access is needed to reduce or inspect the hernial contents. The defect is closed usually using nonabsorbable monofilament sutures, either interrupted or continuous, or a combination; however, many surgeons use mesh, depending on the size and physical demands of the patient. Recurrent hernias often require mesh. The subcutaneous tissues are closed with an absorbable suture and skin closed with a continuous subcuticular suture or staples.

Anatomical Points

The anatomy of the linea alba region is relatively constant. Divarication of the rectus muscles may produce a broad bulge especially evident on lifting the head from the lying position, which is not a hernia, but can appear similar to an epigastric herniation. An epigastric hernia is usually more confined and smaller, and in the relaxed recumbent patient is able to be gently inverted to palpate a distinct edge to the defect and sometimes abdominal contents. It protrudes on coughing (especially

Table 6.1 Surgery for epigastric hernia estimated frequency of complications, risks, and consequences

Complications, risks, and consequences	Estimated frequency
Most significant/serious complications	
Bruising	50–80 %
Bleeding/hematoma formation[a]	5–20 %
Infection	1–5 %
Seroma formation	5–20 %
Rare significant/serious problems	
Suture abscess ± suture sinus[a]	0.1–1 %
Hernia recurrence[a]	0.1–1 %
Laparotomy (bowel injury or adhesion related strangulation)[a]	0.1–1 %
Dehiscence	<0.1 %
Less serious complications	
Pain/discomfort/tenderness	
Acute (<4 weeks)	20–50 %
Chronic (>12 weeks)	0.1–1 %
Scarring	1–5 %
Dimpling/deformity of the skin[a]	1–5 %
Numbness/altered sensation	1–5 %
Drain tube(s)[a]	1–5 %

[a]Dependent on underlying pathology, anatomy, surgical technique, and preferences

when standing), exhibiting a "cough impulse," whereas in divarication the abdominal wall tends to tighten and any "cough impulse" is much less, or absent. Occasionally, an epigastric hernia is irreducible and a mass is palpable often with a narrow (constricting) neck. At operation, the linea alba fibers are often split apart and lie condensed at the edge of the hernial defect (Table 6.1).

Perspective

Most symptomatic epigastric hernias cause discomfort rather than bowel obstruction. Because of the narrow defect in some cases, chronic incarceration of preperitoneal fat is not uncommon, and these herniae are irreducible. The risk of infection is increased when bowel is obstructed. If bowel obstruction is present, the offending loop must be visualized and its viability assessed at the time of repair. This may require extension of the incision or conversion to full laparotomy to assess bowel viability. The usual complications associated with abdominal wall surgery are seen. Monofilament, nonabsorbable suture is usually used to repair the defect. Plastic mesh is sometimes used; however, this slightly increases the risk of foreign body reactions and infection. To date, recurrence rates have not been formally assessed in prospective trials, but are generally considered to be infrequent.

Major Complications

Infections are mainly of skin (*Staphylococcus aureus*) origin; however, bowel derived organisms (*Escherichia coli*; bacteroides sp.; Strep pyogenes) may be caus- ative when bowel is obstructed or breached. Infection often necessitates removal of some, or all, foreign material such as sutures and mesh and may dictate later hernia repair. Infection also increases the risk of suture sinus, **dehiscence**, and hernia recur- rence. **Bleeding** may occur from vessels associated with the edge of the peritoneal hernial sac, and especially from omental vessels that are often thin walled and easily traumatized. Occasionally, mesenteric vessels can be traumatized during reduction of bowel causing bleeding. These situations do not usually present difficulty in obtain- ing control of bleeding. **Bowel Injury** is a potentially serious problem and can occur easily if ischemia and/or infarction of bowel is present. Extension of the incision or midline conventional **laparotomy** is often safest to fully inspect the bowel. Occasionally perforation has occurred and infection is established before surgery. This can present some difficulty with regard to repair using a nonabsorbable suture or mesh. However, mass closure using monofilament sutures is usually satisfactory. Avoidance of mesh, or any foreign material that is more than absolutely necessary for closure, is advisable. Rarely, delayed primary closure is indicated, with subsequent delayed elective hernia repair some months later. **Suture Sinus** may develop as a result of a foreign body reaction to suture material, especially knots, or mesh. Infection can cause, or be secondary to, suture sinuses. When established, a suture sinus will usually only settle after removal of the offending foreign material. However, removal of some of the material may be sufficient, and then the main bulk of material used in the repair can be retained. Sometimes, however, all foreign material has to be removed to heal the sinus and/or infection. There is a small incidence of **hernia recurrence** after repair, and although patients should be warned about this, it is usu- ally not problematic in most cases. **Seroma Formation** produces a lump, which usu- ally resorbes spontaneously and settles and may need needle aspiration drainage(s) to assist this. However, needle aspiration may increase the risk of secondary infection.

Consent and Risk Reduction

Main Points to Explain

- Discomfort
- Bleeding
- Infection
- Bowel perforation
- Recurrent hernia
- Laparotomy
- Further surgery
- Risks without surgery

Surgery for Umbilical/Paraumbilical Hernia

Description

General anesthesia is usually used; however local infiltration and high spinal anesthesia can be used in selected cases, with or without systemic neuroleptic agents. One or multiple defects may be present. The aim of the procedure is to define the sac(s), then excise and repair the defect(s). A transverse skin incision either below or above the umbilicus is usually used. Rarely a longitudinal midline incision is utilized. Umbilical and paraumbilical hernias (UH/PUH) are relatively common surgical problems that spans the ages and sexes in nearly equal frequency. *Umbilical herniae* are through the embryological physiological defect at the umbilical cord where the expanding gut tube herniates and returns to the abdominal cavity by 10 weeks of gestation. Umbilical herniae are common at birth and usually close by the age of 2 years. Many adults have these as persistent umbilical defects, but are never aware of this until pointed out by a surgeon. *Paraumbilical herniae* are usually defined as acquired defects in the abdominal wall cicatrix adjacent to the umbilicus, but many regard this distinction as somewhat artificial. In essence, both umbilical and paraumbilical herniae are managed surgically the same way. The herniae have a peritoneal sac usually containing omentum. Less commonly bowel may herniate, particularly in larger herniae. In obese patients, the diagnosis may be especially difficult. Most UH/PUH are reducible using gentle compression and a finger can often be inserted into the hernial defect inverting the skin and sac to palpate a "cough impulse" as the patient coughs. The hernia is usually rapidly re-created after the examining finger is removed and the patient coughs again. Elective repair is indicated in symptomatic patients; incarceration and bowel obstruction require emergency intervention. Since there is a greater risk of bowel herniation in UH/PUH, than epigastric hernia, there is a tendency to recommend surgical repair for UH/PUH. The sac is defined and excised at the edge of the linea defect, and from the overlying skin of the umbilicus, to expose the contents before reduction. A midline longitudinal incision through the linea alba above and/or below the UH/PUH defect is usual to extend the hernial opening, if better access is needed to reduce or inspect the hernial contents. The defect is closed usually using nonabsorbable monofilament sutures, either interrupted or continuous, or a combination; however, many surgeons use mesh, depending on the size and physical demands of the patient. Recurrent hernias often require mesh. The subcutaneous tissues are closed with an absorbable suture and skin closed with a continuous subcuticular suture or staples.

Anatomical Points

Additional defects should be sought at the time of repair because there may be associated midline abnormalities or fascial defects lateral to the midline at the

Table 6.2 Surgery for umbilical/paraumbilical hernia estimated frequency of complications, risks, and consequences

Complications, risks, and consequences	Estimated frequency
Most significant/serious complications	
Bruising (including minor and severe)	>80 %
Bleeding/hematoma formation[a]	5–20 %
Seroma formation	5–20 %
Infection	1–5 %
Rare significant/serious problems	
Laparotomy (bowel injury or adhesion related strangulation)[a]	0.1–1 %
Hernia recurrence[a] (10 year)	0.1–1 %
Dehiscence	<0.1 %
Less serious complications	
Pain/discomfort/tenderness	
Acute (<4 weeks)	20–50 %
Chronic (>12 weeks)	0.1–1 %
Dimpling/deformity of the Skin[a]	1–5 %
Numbness/altered sensation	1–5 %
Scarring	1–5 %
Suture abscess ± suture sinus[a]	0.1–1 %
Drain tube(s)[a]	1–5 %

[a]Dependent on underlying pathology, anatomy, surgical technique, and preferences

umbilicus. Missing these at the initial operation leads to an apparent increased "recurrence" rate (actually separate herniae). To avoid this event digital or visual exploration of the midline at least 10 cm around the umbilicus is advocated to detect a synchronous herniae; if present, repair is needed to avoid the risk of a "recurrence" (Table 6.2).

Perspective

The complications related to UH/PUH repair are generally not major, but in certain situations infection and bleeding can be problematic. At times, the defect must be enlarged to effect reduction and inspection of the contents and in that situation mesh should be considered an element in the repair. Numbness and injury to nerves is not likely in this procedure given the anatomy and innervation of the central abdominal wall. However, discomfort can persist for some time in some patients and may be a source of dissatisfaction. Occasionally, especially after weight loss, the suture ends or mesh can become palpable and irritating; however, this is partly determined by surgical technique. Repair using laparoscopic techniques produces a different distribution of complications associated with the risks to intra-abdominal organs from laparoscopic entry into the abdomen. Hernia recurrence is related to the quality of the patient's tissues and surgical technique.

Major Complications

Infection is not usually a problem; however, skin organisms predominate unless bowel injury has occurred. The use of mesh or nonabsorbable sutures may engender bacterial colonization and increase the risk of infection slightly. **Wound dehiscence** is rare. **Bleeding** is seldom severe unless an omental or mesenteric vessel is transected, especially at the edge of the peritoneal hernial sac, and from omental vessels that are often thin walled and easily traumatized. The porto-systemic venous anastomoses around the umbilicus can produce annoying bleeding, but in rare patients with portal hypertension, bleeding can be substantial and greater care must be taken. Occasionally, mesenteric vessels can be traumatized during reduction of bowel causing bleeding. These situations do not usually present difficulty in obtaining control of bleeding. **Fluid leakage**, and particularly ascitic leakage is more of a problem in patients with established ascites. **Bowel injury** is a potentially serious problem and can occur easily if ischemia and/or infarction of bowel is present. Extension of the incision or midline conventional **laparotomy** is often safest to fully inspect the bowel, if required. Occasionally perforation has occurred and infection is established before surgery. This can present some difficulty with regard to repair using a nonabsorbable suture or mesh. However, mass closure using monofilament sutures is usually satisfactory. Avoidance of mesh, or any foreign material that is more than absolutely necessary for closure, is advisable in situations of bowel perforation. Rarely, delayed primary closure is indicated, with subsequent delayed elective hernia repair some months later. **Suture Sinus** may develop as a result of a foreign body reaction to suture material, especially knots, or mesh. Infection can cause, or be secondary to, suture sinuses. When established, a suture sinus will usually only settle after removal of the offending foreign material. However, removal of some of the material may be sufficient, and then the main bulk of material used in the repair can be retained. Sometimes, however, all foreign material has to be removed to heal the sinus and/or infection. **Hernia recurrence** rates for these hernia repair complications are rather high and further increased in the presence of obesity. The use of prosthetic mesh in the repair is advocated if the defect exceeds 3 cm in diameter, the tissues are weak or likely to be repeatedly stressed. Placement of the mesh below the rectus fascia and above the peritoneum has been advocated to minimize recurrence, but placement superficial to the fascia is also successful. Weakened tissues are a major reason for initial herniation and also for recurrence.

Consent and Risk Reduction

Main Points to Explain

- Discomfort
- Bleeding
- Infection

- Bowel perforation
- Recurrent hernia
- Laparotomy
- Further surgery
- Risks without surgery

Surgery for Primary Open Inguinal Hernia

Description

Open inguinal hernia repair can be performed under general, local, or regional (spinal or epidural block) anesthesia. The aim is to define and locate the type (direct, indirect, or both) of inguinal hernia and repair it. A lower abdominal or groin transverse incision is often used, however, an oblique incision is sometimes preferred; both afford good access. Inguinal herniae occur through the anterior abdominal wall via the deep inguinal ring (indirect) or a nonphysiological defect in the transversalis fascia medially (direct) or occasionally both (see anatomy). The defect is closed usually using nonabsorbable monofilament sutures, either interrupted or continuous, or a combination; however, many surgeons use mesh, depending on the size and physical demands of the patient. The subcutaneous tissues are closed with an absorbable suture and skin closed with a continuous subcuticular suture or staples.

Anatomical Points

Indirect inguinal herniae occur through the physiological defect at the deep inguinal ring traveling along the spermatic cord in the male, or the "gubernaculum" in the female. Direct inguinal herniae are nonphysiological defects "directly" through the transversalis fascia. Indirect herniae arise laterally, and direct herniae arise medially, to the inferior epigastric vessels; however, the main hernia mass may lie anywhere along the inguinal canal. Indirect herniae may extend into the scrotum. The size of the defect can vary widely for both types of hernia and both may coexist as a complex or "pantaloon" type hernia, protruding either side of the inferior epigastric vessels. The hernial mass comprises a sac containing fluid, peritoneal and/or omental fat, bowel or bladder. Rarely the appendix or ovary may be included. Because direct herniae are more medially placed, bladder is more often included. The position of the ilioinguinal nerve is highly variable sometimes branching early and can be difficult to identify, increasing its risk of injury. Usually, it overlies the spermatic cord, but may be displaced by the hernia. Varicosities of the spermatic (testicular) veins may make dissection of the hernial sac difficult, increasing the risk of bleeding. Chronic scarring of the sac may also distort the anatomy. The cremaster muscle may be extensive, requiring ligation and excision to permit proper access for repair (Table 6.3).

Table 6.3 Surgery for open inguinal hernia estimated frequency of complications, risks, and consequences

Complications, risks, and consequences	Estimated frequency
Most significant/serious complications	
Bruising	50–80 %
Bleeding or hematoma formation[a]	1–5 %
Infection[a]	0.1–1 %
Seroma formation	1–5 %
Numbness/altered sensation	1–5 %
Neural injury[a]	
Ilioinguinal nerve	1–5 %
Iliohypogastric nerve	1–5 %
Hernia recurrence[a] (10 year)	1–5 %
Rare significant/serious problems	
Vascular injury—artery or vein	0.1–1 %
Arterial injury	0.1–1 %
Constriction of femoral vein	<0.1 %
Deep venous thrombosis	0.1–1 %
Suture abscess/granuloma formation ± suture sinus[a]	0.1–1 %
Spermatic cord injury[a]	0.1–1 %
Testicular ischemia, testicular atrophy	0.1–1 %
Testicular necrosis/orchidectomy (rare in repair of primary inguinal hernias)	<0.1 %
Small bowel obstruction	0.1–1 %
Laparotomy (bowel injury or adhesion related strangulation or ischemia)[a]	0.1–1 %
Dehiscence	<0.1 %
Injury to femoral nerve	<0.1 %
Less serious complications	
Pain/discomfort/tenderness (wound/testicular/thigh pain)[a]	
Acute (<4 weeks)	20–50 %
Chronic (>12 weeks)	0.1–1 %
Wound scarring (all)	1–5 %
Dimpling/deformity of the skin[a]	0.1–1 %
Scrotal/labial swelling	5–20 %
Urinary retention	1–5 %
Drain tube(s)[a]	1–5 %

[a]Dependent on underlying pathology, anatomy, surgical technique, and preferences

Perspective

Quantification of the complications associated with open repair of inguinal hernias is difficult for many reasons related to the underreporting of complications as for many surgical procedures. Infection, bleeding, and bowel injury are the major complications of note. Laparotomy for bowel iatrogenic injury is very rare and stoma formation because of this even more rare, but both are reported. It is more commonly associated with bowel incarceration and infarction. Given the number of hernia repairs done annually around the world, and the number of surgeons performing these repairs, it is expected that the results will vary from center to center. A few randomized trials of sufficient size have managed to establish reference values for most of the complications seen in open groin hernia repair. Of course, the wide variety of repairs available will not have the same complication rates; however, some complications will be common and others unique to the specific repair. Hence the rather broad range of frequencies for each of the "common" complications noted. Some readers will perceive some of the values to be too high based on their experience. Many of the complications are indeed rare and clearly relate to the specific technique or repair employed. Modern surgical training has all but eliminated the spermatic cord, testicular and vascular injury noted in the past, reducing these to the relatively rare range when in the past these figures were considerably higher. More modern studies have looked at post-hernia repair pain, now reported as high as 50 % in some prospective studies; it is considered a major issue. Indeed, there appears to be a significant increase in the incidence of post-repair chronic pain that is not entirely understood and may be related to the use of prosthetic mesh as the primary basis for the repair. Only recently true recurrence rates have been appreciated for the various anterior repairs and they all are in the 1–2 % range, independent of technique. When discussing recurrence rates it is important to note that many patients with recurrence appear years after the repair and recurrence rates at 10 and 20 years are yet to be established for many of the more common repairs in use today. Acute hernia repair failure, within days to weeks is likely to be underreported. With the introduction of the tension free approach to the repair of groin hernia, acute failures are rare. There is variation depending on the individual, center or site reporting their experience; however, there is an apparent increase in the incidence of chronic pain associated with this repair dependent on the intensity of investigation.

Major Complications

Infection is chiefly from skin (*S. aureus*) origin. Bowel derived organisms (*E. coli*; bacteroides sp.; Strep pyogenes) may be causative when bowel is obstructed or breached. Infection often necessitates removal of some, or all, foreign material such as sutures and mesh and may dictate later hernia repair. Infection also increases the risk of suture sinus, **dehiscence**, and hernia recurrence. **Bleeding** may occur from vessels associated with the edge of the peritoneal hernial sac, including the inferior epigastric vessels, outside the sac. Within the sac, the omental vessels are often thin walled and easily traumatized and occasionally mesenteric vessels can be traumatized during reduction of bowel, causing bleeding. Testicular or cremasteric vessels may also bleed. These situations do not usually present difficulty in obtaining control of bleeding. **Bowel Injury** is a potentially serious problem and can occur easily if ischemia and/or infarction of bowel is present due to incarceration and strangulation. Conventional midline **laparotomy**, or perhaps lateral incision of the deep ring, is often safest to fully inspect the bowel, if needed. Occasionally, perforation has

occurred before surgery and infection is established. This can present some difficulty with regard to repair using any nonabsorbable suture. Avoidance of mesh, or
any foreign material that is more than absolutely necessary for closure, is advisable.
Delayed primary closure may be then indicated, with subsequent delayed elective
hernia repair some months later. However, in special cases mass closure using
monofilament sutures might still be performed. **Suture Sinus** may develop as a
result of a foreign body reaction to suture material, especially knots, or mesh.
Infection may either cause, or be secondary to suture sinuses. When established, a
suture sinus will usually only settle after removal of the offending foreign material.
However, removal of only some of the material may be required and frequently the
main bulk of material used in the repair can be retained if granulation of tissue
occurs over the mesh. Sometimes, however, all foreign material has to be removed
to heal the sinus and/or infection. There is a small incidence of **hernia recurrence**
after repair, and although patients should be warned about this, it is usually not
problematic in most cases. The recurrence rate increases with the time observed and
after infection-related hernia complications.

Consent and Risk Reduction

Main Points to Explain

- Discomfort
- Bleeding
- Infection
- Bowel perforation
- Recurrent hernia
- Laparotomy
- Further surgery
- Risks without surgery

Surgery for Recurrent Open Inguinal Hernia

Description

Recurrent open inguinal hernia repair can be performed under general, local, or
regional (spinal or epidural block) anesthesia. The aim is to define and repair the
recurrent hernia, usually using monofilament suture material or mesh. A lower
abdominal or groin transverse or oblique incision is often used, and typically the old
scar from the previous repair(s) is excised, if that is appropriate. Recurrent inguinal
herniae can occur through the anterior abdominal wall via the same or a different

defect at the deep inguinal ring (indirect) or in the transversalis fascia (direct) (see anatomy). Direct inguinal hernia "recurrence" is more common. Recurrent indirect inguinal herniae after a technically correct ligation of an indirect sac and repair should be very rare; however, occasionally an indirect sac is not detected at operation for a direct hernia. Recurrence of a direct hernia at the medial end of an indirect hernia repair is the commonest reported recurrent inguinal hernia site. This probably arises from failure to continue the repair sufficiently far enough medially, and/or recurrently weakened tissues. The defect is closed usually using nonabsorbable monofilament sutures, either interrupted or continuous, or a combination; however, many surgeons use mesh, depending on the size and physical demands of the patient. Recurrent hernias often require mesh. The subcutaneous tissues are closed with an absorbable suture and skin closed with a continuous subcuticular suture or staples.

Anatomical Points

Recurrent inguinal herniae usually occur directly through a nonphysiological defect in the transversalis fascia (direct hernia), but can occur through the physiological defect at the deep inguinal ring (indirect hernia) traveling along the spermatic cord in the male, or the gubernaculum in the female. Indirect herniae arise laterally and direct herniae arise medially to the inferior epigastric vessels; however, the main hernia mass may lie anywhere along the inguinal canal. Indirect herniae may extend into the scrotum. The size of the defect can vary widely for both types of hernia and both may coexist as a complex or "pantaloon" type hernia, either side of the inferior epigastric vessels. The hernial mass comprises a sac containing fluid, peritoneal and/or omental fat, bowel or bladder. Rarely the appendix or ovary may be included. Because direct herniae are more medially placed, bladder is more often included. The position of the ilioinguinal nerve is highly variable and this may branch early and can be difficult to identify, increasing the risk of injury, especially so for recurrent herniae due to scarring. Usually it overlies the spermatic cord, but may be displaced by the hernia or scar tissue. Varicosities of the spermatic (testicular) veins may make dissection of the hernial sac difficult, and entrapment of testicular vessels in scar tissue can increase the risk bleeding and testicular ischemia. Chronic scarring from previous surgery may also distort the anatomy. The cremaster muscle may be extensive, requiring ligation and excision to permit proper access for repair (Table 6.4).

Perspective

There are many potential complications associated with open repair for recurrent groin herniae. Many are related to the specific techniques and approaches used for both the original and recurrent hernia repairs. Anterior or posterior/pre-peritoneal approaches with or without mesh can be used. Previous anterior repairs often leave

Table 6.4 Surgery for recurrent open inguinal hernia estimated frequency of complications, risks, and consequences

Complications, risks, and consequences	Estimated frequency
Most significant/serious complications	
Bruising	50–80 %
Bleeding/hematoma formation[a]	1–5 %
Infection[a]	0.1–1 %
Seroma formation	5–20 %
Numbness/altered sensation	1–5 %
Neural injury[a]	
Ilioinguinal nerve	5–20 %
Iliohypogastric nerve	5–20 %
Ilioinguinal, iliohypogastric, genitofemoral nerve paresthesia[a]	20–50 %
Hernia recurrence[a] (10 year)	1–5 %
Rare significant/serious problems	
Femoral nerve paresthesia (if femoral nerve block used)[a]	0.1–1 %
Vascular injury—artery or vein	0.1–1 %
Constriction of femoral vein	<0.1 %
Arterial injury	0.1–1 %
Deep venous thrombosis	0.1–1 %
Suture abscess/granuloma formation ± suture sinus[a]	0.1–1 %
Spermatic cord injury[a]	0.1–1 %
Testicular ischemia, testicular atrophy	0.1–1 %
Testicular necrosis/orchidectomy (rare in repair of primary inguinal hernias)	<0.1 %
Small bowel obstruction	0.1–1 %
Laparotomy (bowel injury or adhesion related strangulation or ischemia)[a]	0.1–1 %
Fecal fistula	<0.1 %
Urinary fistula	<0.1 %
Dehiscence	<0.1 %
Injury to femoral nerve	<0.1 %
Less serious complications	
Pain/discomfort/tenderness (wound/testicular/thigh pain)[a]	
Acute (<4 weeks)	20–50 %
Chronic (>12 weeks)	0.1–1 %
Scrotal/labial swelling	5–20 %
Wound scarring	1–5 %
Urinary retention	1–5 %
Dimpling/deformity of the skin[a]	1–5 %
Wound scarring	1–5 %
Drain tube(s)[a]	1–5 %

[a]Dependent on underlying pathology, anatomy, surgical technique, and preferences

scarring making a repeat anterior approach more dangerous for injury to the testicular vessels and vas deferens. The posterior approach often offers better-defined tissue planes and minimal scarring, reducing risk. The posterior approach has the advantage of dissecting through relatively unscarred tissues. In 800 cases, the recurrence rate for first-time recurrent groin hernia was 1.6 %, and for multiply recurrent defects about 3.5 % at 5 years. Similar results have been reported recently from randomized trials. Surgeon's experience is a key factor in minimizing complications associated with the repair of any recurrent hernia independent of the approach selected. Working in the pre-peritoneal space demands the experience and an appreciation of the anatomy in order to effect a complete repair of all the defects found. Injury to peripheral nerves, ilioinguinal, iliohypogastric, and iliofemoral is seen more frequently with the anterior repair of recurrent hernias. Chronic groin pain after surgery for recurrent inguinal herniae is not uncommon. In a detailed analysis of recurrent hernia defects defined at the time of pre-peritoneal repair, 15 % of the defects were classified as complex or multiple, often unsuspected preoperatively, supporting the posterior approach for repair of these hernias. The posterior approach affords complete visual access to the entire inguinal floor and thus allows definition of all defects so that complete repair is possible. There are increased risks of injury to bowel, bladder, or vessels if one is not familiar with the anatomy. The laparoscopic approach to the repair of recurrent groin hernia—predicated on the posterior approach—has a slightly higher reported incidence of early failure and nerve and vessel injury. Avoiding the major complications in the repair of recurrent groin hernias reflects training, care, experience, and judgement, with each of the latter a function of the former.

Major Complications

Infection is mainly of skin (*S. aureus*) origin. Bowel derived organisms (*E. coli*; bacteroides sp.; Strep pyogenes) may be causative when bowel is obstructed or breached. Infection often necessitates removal of some, or all, foreign material such as sutures and mesh and may dictate later hernia repair. Infection also increases the risk of suture sinus, dehiscence, and hernia recurrence. **Bleeding** may occur from vessels associated with the edge of the peritoneal hernial sac, including the inferior epigastric vessels, outside the sac. Within the sac, the omental vessels are often thin walled and easily traumatized and occasionally mesenteric vessels can be traumatized during reduction of bowel, causing bleeding. Testicular or cremasteric vessels may also bleed. These situations do not usually present difficulty in obtaining control of bleeding. **Bowel injury** is a potentially serious problem and can occur easily if ischemia and/or infarction of bowel is present due to incarceration and strangulation. Conventional midline **laparotomy**, or perhaps lateral incision of the deep ring, is often safest to fully inspect the bowel. Occasionally perforation has occurred before surgery and infection is established. This can present some difficulty with regard to repair using any nonabsorbable suture. Avoidance of mesh, or any foreign material that is more than absolutely necessary for closure, is advisable. Delayed primary closure may be then indicated, with subsequent delayed elective hernia repair some months later. However, in special cases mass closure using monofilament sutures might still be performed. **Testicular injury** is not uncommon during recurrent inguinal hernia repair, especially with a repeated anterior approach, due to dense scar tissue and/or mesh entrapping the testicular blood supply and cord. Vascular injury causes testicular ischemia, and if sufficient may necessitate orchidectomy. **Suture sinus** may develop as a result of a foreign body reaction to suture material, especially knots, or mesh. Infection may either cause, or be secondary to suture sinuses. When established, a suture sinus will usually only settle after removal of the offending foreign material. However, removal of only some of the material may be required and frequently the main bulk of material used in the repair can be retained if granulation of tissue occurs over the mesh. Sometimes, however, all foreign material has to be removed to heal the sinus and/or infection. There is a recognized incidence of **hernia recurrence** after repeat hernia repair, and although patients should be warned about this, it is usually not problematic in most cases. The recurrence rate is time dependent. The factors that have lead to one recurrence, such as weak tissues may contribute to further recurrences.

Consent and Risk Reduction

Main Points to Explain

- Discomfort
- Bleeding
- Infection
- Bowel perforation
- Recurrent hernia
- Laparotomy
- Testicular injury/removal
- Further surgery
- Risks without surgery

Surgery for Laparoscopic Hernia Repair (Pre-Peritoneal Approach)

Description

Laparoscopic TEP approach to inguinal hernia repair is performed under general anesthesia. Inguinal herniae occur through the anterior abdominal wall via the deep inguinal ring or a nonphysiological defect in the transversalis fascia (see anatomy). Laparoscopic approaches are also increasingly used for recurrent or bilateral hernia repairs.

Anatomical Points

Indirect inguinal herniae occur through the physiological defect at the deep inguinal ring traveling along the spermatic cord in the male, or the gubernaculum in the female. Direct inguinal herniae are nonphysiological defects "directly" through the transversalis fascia. Indirect herniae arise laterally and direct herniae arise medially to the inferior epigastric vessels; however, the main hernia mass may lie anywhere along the inguinal canal. Indirect herniae may extend into the scrotum. The size of the defect can vary widely for both types of hernia and both may coexist as a complex or "pantaloon" type hernia, protruding either side of the inferior epigastric vessels. The hernial mass comprises a sac containing fluid, peritoneal and/or omental fat, bowel or bladder. Rarely the appendix or ovary may be included. Because direct herniae are more medially placed, bladder is more often included. Varicosities of the spermatic (testicular) veins may make dissection of the hernial sac difficult, increasing the risk of bleeding. Chronic scarring of the sac may also distort the anatomy. Adequate definition of the anatomy is important (Table 6.5).

Perspective

The TEP "repair" reinforces the extraperitoneal (pre-peritoneal) aspect of the posterior wall of the inguinal canal and therefore associated with complications related to "technical and anatomic" issues. In general, the complications are similar in type and frequency to the TAPP repair. Knowledge of the anatomy and the variations commonly seen is helpful in minimizing nerve and vessel injury, especially to the retroperitoneal structures in the TEP approach. Vascular and bowel injury are more likely with these repairs and there is an increased, yet still low level of risk for bladder injury. It must be noted that the potential intra-abdominal complications associated with laparoscopic access add a new dimension of complications not usually associated with hernia repair. These are more frequent in the TAPP approach it being trans-peritoneal access, thus putting the intra-abdominal contents at increased risk for injury. Laparoscopic repairs are rooted in information gleaned from the development of the open pre-peritoneal repair of groin hernia. Recurrence rates are low, but still definable and may relate to the "learning curve" of experience, as would any newly acquired procedure. Bowel and bladder injury are more common when the peritoneal cavity is inadvertently entered, but may reflect the surgeon's experience and theoretically should be minimized with more experience. However, there is an intrinsic complication rate associated with the laparoscopic approach that may never be eliminated, perhaps at best minimized by experience.

Table 6.5 Surgery for laparoscopic (pre-peritoneal approach) estimated frequency of complications, risks, and consequences

Complications, risks, and consequences	Estimated frequency
Most significant/serious complications	
Bleeding/hematoma formation[a]	1–5 %
Hernia recurrence[a] (5 year)	1–5 %
Injury to ilioinguinal nerve	1–5 %
Spermatic cord injury (overall)[a]	1–5 %
Testicular ischemia, testicular atrophy	1–5 %
Testicular necrosis/orchidectomy (rare in repair of primary inguinal hernias)	0.1–1 %
Urinary retention	1–5 %
Rare significant/serious problems	
Infection[a]	0.1–1 %
Laparotomy (bowel injury or adhesion related strangulation or ischemia)[a]	0.1–1 %
Conversion to open surgical procedure (inclusive loss of pneumo-pre peritoneum)	0.1–1 %
Vascular injury—artery or vein (overall)[a]	0.1–1 %
Constriction of femoral vein	
Arterial injury	
Deep venous thrombosis[a]	0.1–1 %
Injury to femoral nerve	0.1–1 %
Small bowel obstruction	<0.1 %
Dehiscence	<0.1 %
Gas embolus	<0.1 %
Mortality[a]	<0.1 %
Less serious complications	
Pain/discomfort/tenderness (wound/testicular/thigh pain)[a]	
Acute (<4 weeks)	20–50 %
Chronic (>12 weeks)	0.1–1 %
Bruising	20–50 %
Seroma formation	1–5 %
Numbness/altered sensation	1–5 %
Functional impairment[a]	1–5 %
Scrotal/labial swelling	1–5 %
Suture abscess/granuloma formation ± suture sinus	0.1–1 %
Wound scarring	1–5 %
Dimpling/deformity of the skin	1–5 %
Port-site hernia formation	<0.1 %
Drain tube(s)[a]	1–5 %

[a]Dependent on underlying pathology, anatomy, surgical technique, and preferences

Major Complications

The main **infections** are of skin (*S. aureus*) origin. Bowel derived organisms (*E. coli*; bacteroides sp.; Strep pyogenes) may be causative when bowel is obstructed or breached. Infection often necessitates removal of some, or all, foreign material such as sutures and mesh and may dictate later hernia repair. Infection also increases the risk of suture sinus, dehiscence, and hernia recurrence. **Bleeding** may occur from vessels associated with the abdominal wall, edge of the peritoneal hernial sac, including the inferior epigastric vessels, outside the sac. Within the sac, the omental vessels are often thin walled and easily traumatized and occasionally mesenteric vessels can be traumatized during reduction of bowel, causing bleeding. Testicular or cremasteric vessels may also bleed. These situations do not usually present difficulty in obtaining control of bleeding. Rare, catastrophic hemorrhage from direct puncture of a major vessel (aorta or iliac) is reported, but may be minimized by careful dissection in the extraperitoneal plane. **Bowel injury** is a potentially serious problem and can occur easily if ischemia and/or infarction of bowel is present due to incarceration and strangulation. Conventional midline **laparotomy**, or perhaps lateral incision of the deep ring, is often safest to fully inspect the bowel. Occasionally perforation has occurred before surgery and infection is established. This can present some difficulty with regard to repair using any nonabsorbable suture. Avoidance of mesh, or any foreign material that is more than absolutely necessary for closure, is advisable. Delayed primary closure may be then indicated, with subsequent delayed elective hernia repair some months later. However, in special cases mass closure using monofilament sutures might still be performed. **Bowel obstruction** may occur after inadvertent intra-abdominal entry, and cases have been reported with trans-abdominal laparoscopic hernia repair. However, this is still an uncommon event on available evidence. **Testicular injury** is not uncommon during recurrent inguinal hernia repair, due to dense scar tissue and/or mesh entrapping the testicular blood supply and cord. Vascular injury causes testicular ischemia, and if sufficient may necessitate orchidectomy. **Suture sinus** may develop as a result of a foreign body reaction to suture material, especially knots, or mesh. Infection may either cause, or be secondary to suture sinuses. When established, a suture sinus will usually only settle after removal of the offending foreign material. However, removal of only some of the material may be required and frequently the main bulk of material used in the repair can be retained if granulation of tissue occurs over the mesh. Sometimes, however, all foreign material has to be removed to heal the sinus and/or infection. There is a recognized incidence of **hernia recurrence** after primary or repeat hernia repair, and although patients should be warned about this, it is usually not problematic in most cases. The recurrence rate is time dependent. The factors that have led to one recurrence, such as weak tissues may contribute to further recurrences. The long-term recurrence rates for laparoscopic hernia repairs are not yet available, but shorter-term rates are comparable with open procedures. **Gas embolism** is a rare, but catastrophic event arising from entry of insufflation gas (CO_2) into vessels usually within the abdominal wall, occurring from direct puncture by a Veress needle. **Port-site hernias** are reported for most laparoscopic abdominal procedures and are more common with larger incisions and entry into the peritoneal cavity. **Chronic wound pain** is reported with laparoscopic approaches and has been suggested to be due to stapling, clips or sutures, and scarring from surgery. Early studies have shown that it is perhaps more common than with open approaches; however, this may be experience dependant.

Consent and Risk Reduction

Main Points to Explain

- Discomfort
- Bleeding
- Infection
- Bowel perforation
- Recurrent hernia
- Laparotomy
- Further surgery
- Risks without surgery

Surgery for Laparoscopic Hernia Repair (Intra/Trans-Peritoneal Approach)

Description

TAPP laparoscopic approach to inguinal hernia repair is usually performed under general anesthesia with muscle relaxation. Inguinal herniae occur through the anterior abdominal wall via the deep inguinal ring or a nonphysiological defect in the transversalis fascia (see anatomy). Laparoscopic approaches are also increasingly used for recurrent hernia repairs, sometimes these are via entry to the peritoneal cavity.

Anatomical Points

Indirect inguinal herniae occur through the physiological defect at the deep inguinal ring traveling along the spermatic cord in the male, or the gubernaculum in the female. Direct inguinal herniae are nonphysiological defects "directly" through the transversalis fascia. Indirect herniae arise laterally and direct herniae arise medially to the inferior epigastric vessels; however, the main hernia mass may lie anywhere along the inguinal canal. Indirect herniae may extend into the scrotum. The size of the defect can vary widely for both types of hernia and both may coexist as a complex or "pantaloon" type hernia, protruding either side of the inferior epigastric vessels. The hernial mass comprises a sac containing fluid, peritoneal and/or omental fat, bowel or bladder. Rarely the appendix or ovary may be included. Because direct herniae are more medially placed, bladder is more often included. Varicosities of the spermatic (testicular) veins may make dissection of the hernial sac difficult, increasing the risk of bleeding. Chronic scarring of the sac may also distort the anatomy. Adequate definition of the anatomy is important (Table 6.6).

Table 6.6 Surgery for laparoscopic (intra/trans-peritoneal approach) estimated frequency of complications, risks, and consequences

Complications, risks, and consequences	Estimated frequency
Most significant/serious complications	
Bleeding or hematoma formation[a]	1–5 %
Hernia recurrence[a] (5 year)	1–5 %
Injury to ilioinguinal nerve	1–5 %
Spermatic cord injury (overall)[a]	1–5 %
Testicular ischemia, testicular atrophy	1–5 %
Testicular necrosis/orchidectomy (rare in repair of primary inguinal hernias)	0.1–1 %
Urinary retention	1–5 %
Rare significant/serious problems	
Infection[a]	0.1–1 %
Small bowel obstruction[a]	0.1–1 %
Laparotomy (bowel injury or adhesion related strangulation or ischemia)[a]	0.1–1 %
Injury to femoral nerve	0.1–1 %
Vascular injury—artery or vein (overall)[a]	0.1–1 %
Constriction of femoral vein	
Arterial injury	
Conversion to open surgical procedure (inclusive loss of pneumo-peritoneum)[a]	0.1–1 %
Deep venous thrombosis[a]	0.1–1 %
Dehiscence[a]	<0.1 %
Gas embolus	<0.1 %
Mortality[a]	<0.1 %
Less serious complications	
Pain/discomfort/tenderness (wound/testicular/thigh pain)[a]	
Acute (<4 weeks)	20–50 %
Chronic (>12 weeks)	0.1–1 %
Numbness/altered sensation	1–5 %
Bruising	20–50 %
Functional impairment[a]	1–5 %
Scrotal/labial swelling	1–5 %
Seroma formation	1–5 %
Suture abscess/granuloma formation ± suture sinus	0.1–1 %
Wound scarring	1–5 %
Dimpling/deformity of the skin	1–5 %
Port-site hernia formation	<0.1 %
Drain tube(s)[a]	1–5 %

[a]Dependent on underlying pathology, anatomy, surgical technique, and preferences

Perspective

The TAPP "repair" is to the posterior wall of the inguinal canal and therefore associated with complications related to "technical and anatomic" issues. In general the complications are similar in type and frequency to the TEP repair. Knowledge of the anatomy and the variations commonly seen is helpful in minimizing nerve and vessel injury, especially to intra-abdominal structures in the TAPP approach. Vascular and bowel injury are more likely with these repairs and there is an increased, yet still low level of risk for bladder injury. It must be noted that the intra-abdominal complications associated with laparoscopic access add a new dimension of complications not usually associated with hernia repair. These are more frequent in the TAPP approach it being trans-peritoneal access, thus putting the intra-abdominal contents at increased risk for injury. Laparoscopic repairs are rooted in information gleaned from the development of the open pre-peritoneal repair of groin hernia. Recurrence rates are low but still definable and may relate to the "learning curve" of experience, as would any newly acquired procedure. Bowel and bladder injury are more common with trans-peritoneal approaches, but may reflect the surgeon's experience and theoretically should be minimized with more experience. However, there is an intrinsic complication rate associated with the laparoscopic approach that may never be eliminated, perhaps at best minimized by experience.

Major Complications

The main **infections** are of skin (*S. aureus*) origin. Bowel derived organisms (*E. coli*; bacteroides sp.; Strep pyogenes) may be causative when bowel is obstructed or breached. Infection often necessitates removal of some or all foreign material such as sutures and mesh and may dictate later hernia repair. Infection also increases the risk of suture sinus, dehiscence, and hernia recurrence. **Bleeding** may occur from vessels associated with the abdominal wall, edge of the peritoneal hernial sac, including the inferior epigastric vessels, outside the sac. Within the sac, the omental vessels are often thin walled and easily traumatized and occasionally mesenteric vessels can be traumatized during reduction of bowel, causing bleeding. Testicular or cremasteric vessels may also bleed. These situations do not usually present difficulty in obtaining control of bleeding. Rare, catastrophic hemorrhage from **direct vascular injury** to a major vessel (aorta or iliac) is reported, but may be minimized by careful, open entry into the abdomen. **Bowel injury** is a potentially serious problem and can occur easily if ischemia and/or infarction of bowel is present due to incarceration and strangulation. Conventional midline **laparotomy**, or perhaps lateral incision of the deep ring, is often safest to fully inspect the bowel. Occasionally perforation has occurred before surgery and infection is established. This can present some difficulty with regard to repair using any nonabsorbable suture. Avoidance of mesh, or any foreign material that is more than absolutely necessary for closure, is advisable. Delayed primary closure may be then indicated, with subsequent delayed elective hernia repair some months later. However, in special cases mass closure using monofilament sutures might still be performed. **Bowel Obstruction** is more common with intra-abdominal surgery, and cases have been reported with trans-abdominal laparoscopic hernia repair. However, this is still an uncommon event on available evidence. **Testicular injury** is not uncommon during recurrent inguinal hernia repair, due to dense scar tissue and/or mesh entrapping the testicular blood supply and cord. Vascular injury causes testicular ischemia, and if sufficient may necessitate orchidectomy. **Suture sinus** may develop as a result of a foreign body reaction to suture material, especially knots, or mesh. Infection may either cause, or be secondary to suture sinuses. When established, a suture sinus will usually only settle after removal of the offending foreign material. However, removal of only some of the material may be required and frequently the main bulk of material used in the repair can be retained if granulation of tissue occurs over the mesh. Sometimes, however, all foreign material has to be removed to heal the sinus and/or infection. There is a recognized incidence of **hernia recurrence** after primary or repeat hernia repair, and although patients should be warned about this, it is usually not problematic in most cases. The recurrence rate is time dependent. The factors that have led to one recurrence, such as weak tissues, may contribute to further recurrences. The long-term recurrence rates for laparoscopic hernia repairs are not yet available, but shorter-term rates are comparable with open procedures. **Port-site hernias** are reported for most laparoscopic abdominal procedures and are more common with larger incisions and entry into the peritoneal cavity. **Gas embolism** is a rare, but catastrophic event arising from entry of insufflation gas (CO_2) into vessels usually within the abdominal wall, occurring from direct puncture by a Veress needle, when used. **Chronic wound pain** is reported with laparoscopic approaches and has been suggested to be due to stapling, clips or sutures, and scarring from surgery. Early studies have shown that it is perhaps more common than with open approaches; however, this may be experience dependent.

Consent and Risk Reduction

Main Points to Explain

- Discomfort
- Bleeding
- Infection
- Bowel perforation
- Recurrent hernia
- Laparotomy
- Further surgery
- Risks without surgery

Surgery for Femoral Hernia Repair

Description

Open femoral hernia repair can be performed under general, local, or regional (spinal or epidural block) anesthesia. Femoral herniae occur through the lower anterior abdominal wall through the widened physiological femoral ring and canal into the antero-medial thigh (see anatomy). There are three common operative approaches used for femoral hernia repair: (1) high (McEvedy) approach using a transverse or vertical muscle cutting para-rectus, or lower midline laparotomy incision and a trans- or pre-peritoneal dissection, (2) inguinal (Lotheissen) approach, via an incision through the posterior wall of the inguinal canal transversalis fascia, with a pre- or trans-peritoneal dissection, and (3) the lower (Lockwood) approach, defining the hernial sac from below and externally. The precise risk and nature of the complications are largely determined by the operative approach, the anatomy, hernial size, and the presence of obstruction or not.

Anatomical Points

Femoral herniae occur through the physiological defect at the femoral ring forming a sac protruding into the femoral canal and traveling along the medial aspect of the femoral vein into the thigh. The size of the defect can vary widely, as can the size of the mass and its contents. Femoral herniae are more common in females. The hernial mass comprises a sac containing fluid, peritoneal and/or omental fat, sometimes with small bowel, bladder, or rarely other organs such as the appendix, ovary or parts of the large bowel. Chronic scarring of the sac may also distort the anatomy. In 1/3 of people an "abnormal" obturator artery (obturator) travels from the inferior epigastric artery to reach the obturator foramen either lateral (90 %) or medial (10 % cases) to the femoral canal. In either case, it is more vulnerable during surgery for a femoral hernia repair. The anatomical structures at risk during surgery for femoral hernia repair are determined largely by the operative approach selected (Table 6.7).

Perspective

Many of the complications associated with femoral hernia surgery relate to the population of generally older women who present with incarceration or bowel obstruction, necessitating an emergency operation in a rather high-risk patient. A generally accepted surgical maxim is that an elective procedure is safer in terms of morbidity and mortality—and the incidence of complications—than the same operation done as an emergency. Thus for femoral hernia the complications observed must be

Table 6.7 Surgery for femoral hernia estimated frequency of complications, risks, and consequences

Complications, risks, and consequences	Estimated frequency
Most significant/serious complications	
Bleeding/hematoma formation[a]	1–5 %
Neural injury	
Obturator nerve	0.1–1 %
Iliohypogastric nerve (high approaches only)	1–5 %
Femoral nerve	<0.1 %
Urinary retention[b]	1–5 %
Small bowel obstruction[a]	1–5 %
Hernia recurrence[a] (10 year)	0.1–1 %
Rare significant/serious problems	
Infection	0.1–1[a] %
Deep venous thrombosis[a]	0.1–1 %
Laparotomy (bowel injury or adhesion related strangulation or ischemia)[a]	0.1–1 %
Vascular injury—artery or vein	0.1–1 %
Constriction of femoral vein	0.1–1 %
Arterial injury	0.1–1 %
Injury to abnormal obturator artery	1–5 %
Dehiscence	<0.1 %
Injury to femoral nerve[a]	<0.1 %
Less serious complications	
Pain/discomfort/tenderness (wound/testicular/thigh pain)[a]	
Acute (<4 weeks)	20–50 %
Chronic (>12 weeks)	0.1–1 %
Numbness/altered sensation (overall)[a]	1–5 %
Bruising	50–80 %
Seroma formation	1–5 %
Scrotal/labial swelling	5–20 %
Suture abscess/granuloma formation ± suture sinus[a]	0.1–1 %
Wound scarring (all)	1–5 %
Dimpling/deformity of the skin	1–5 %
Drain tube(s)[a]	1–5 %

[a]Dependent on underlying pathology, anatomy, surgical technique, and preferences
[b]Almost exclusively in males

differentiated between those associated with a physiologically compromised patient and those directly related to the hernia and its repair. As in all of the other hernia repairs there are general "technically related" complications and those related to specific procedures per se. Anterior, posterior, and infra-ligamentous approaches each has complications specifically associated with femoral hernia repair.

Significant complications are more likely to be nerve or vessel injury given the proximity of the large vessels and cutaneous nerves in this area. Compromise of femoral venous flow is a potentially serious complication of femoral hernia repair independent of approach, and care should be exercised to minimize compression of the femoral vein during the repair to minimize the risk of venous stasis, thrombosis, and possible pulmonary embolism. The posterior pre- or trans-peritoneal approach is "ideal" for the repair of any femoral hernia, elective or emergency and is recommended, especially if bowel entrapment is suspected. Formal laparotomy may be required. Quantification of the complications associated with femoral hernia repair is difficult for many reasons related to the underreporting of complications as for many surgical procedures. Infection, bleeding, and bowel injury are the major complications of note. Many of the complications are indeed rare and clearly relate to the specific technique or repair employed.

Major Complications

The main **infections** are of skin (*S. aureus*) origin. Bowel derived organisms (*E. coli*; bacteroides sp.; Strep pyogenes) may be causative when bowel is obstructed or breached. Infection often necessitates removal of some or all foreign materials such as sutures and mesh and may dictate later hernia repair. Infection also increases the risk of suture sinus, dehiscence, and hernia recurrence. **Bleeding** may occur from vessels associated with the edge of the peritoneal hernial sac, including the inferior epigastric vessels and an abnormal obturator artery (when present), outside the sac. Within the sac, the omental vessels are often thin walled and easily traumatized and occasionally mesenteric vessels can be traumatized during reduction of bowel, causing bleeding. These situations do not usually present difficulty in obtaining control of bleeding. **Bowel injury** is a potentially serious problem and can occur easily if ischemia and/or infarction of bowel is present due to incarceration and strangulation. Conventional midline **laparotomy**, or extension of a lower abdominal muscle cutting incision, is often safest to fully inspect the bowel. Occasionally perforation has occurred before surgery and infection is established. This can present some difficulty with regard to repair using any nonabsorbable suture. Avoidance of mesh, or any foreign material that is more than absolutely necessary for closure, is advisable. Delayed primary closure may be then indicated, with subsequent delayed elective hernia repair some months later. However, in special cases mass closure using monofilament sutures might still be performed. **Suture sinus** may develop as a result of a foreign body reaction to suture material, especially knots, or mesh. Infection may either cause, or be secondary to suture sinuses. When established, a suture sinus will usually only settle after removal of the offending foreign material. However, removal of only some of the material may be required and frequently the main bulk of material used in the repair can be retained if granulation of tissue occurs over the mesh. Sometimes, however, all foreign material has to be removed to heal the sinus and/or infection. There is a small incidence of **hernia recurrence** after repair, and although patients should be warned about this, it is usually not problematic in most cases. The recurrence rate increases with the time observed. **Femoral vein compression** is a possible complication if the femoral canal defect is closed too tightly after reduction of the hernia mass. If the venous stasis occurs, thrombosis and pulmonary embolism may ensue, with serious associated risks.

Consent and Risk Reduction

Main Points to Explain

- Discomfort
- Bleeding
- Infection
- Bowel perforation
- Recurrent hernia
- Laparotomy
- Further surgery
- Risks without surgery

Surgery for Small Incisional Hernia

Description

General anesthesia is usually used; however, local infiltration and occasionally high spinal anesthesia can be used in selected cases, with or without neuroleptic agents. Incisional hernia is a relatively common surgical problem. It typically occurs through a defect in a previous scar allowing abdominal contents to protrude, sometimes containing peritoneum and shows as a bulge, emphasized by coughing. The contents are often pre-peritoneal fat, occasionally omentum and less commonly bowel within a peritoneal sac. It is observed in all ages and both genders almost equally. In obese patients, the diagnosis may be especially difficult. Elective repair is indicated in symptomatic patients; incarceration and bowel obstruction require emergency intervention. Non-operative reduction may be useful to reduce urgency if the period of irreducibility is less than 4 or so hours, depending on the degree of ischemia. Incision/excision of the previous scar is usually appropriate for access, however, a separate longitudinal, midline or transverse skin incision may be used. The sac is defined and excised at the edge of the defect to expose the contents before reduction. An incision through the edge of the defect may be used if better access is needed to reduce or inspect the hernial contents. Occasionally, the hernia is multi-loculated, necessitating more dissection, which usually increases the risk of complications.

Anatomical Points

The anatomy of the region of the previous incision and the contents usually determine the nature and risk of complications. Divarication of the rectus muscles may produce a broad bulge especially evident on lifting the head from the lying position, potentially appearing similar to a midline incisional hernia. In the relaxed recumbent patient, an incisional hernia can often be gently inverted to palpate a distinct edge to the defect and sometimes abdominal contents. It protrudes on coughing (especially when standing), exhibiting a "cough impulse," whereas in divarication the abdominal wall tends to tighten and any "cough impulse" is much less, or absent. Occasionally, an incisional hernia is irreducible and a mass is palpable often with a narrow (constricting) neck. The hernia may protrude through all layers of the abdominal wall, producing the "classical" signs of an incisional hernia. Not infrequently the incisional hernia lies between musculo-fascial layers, where the signs may be less prominent, and the hernia not as easily palpated. At operation, the sac and edge of the defect must be anatomically dissected and defined. Multiple hernial openings are not infrequent making the sac irregular in shape, with adhesions tethering bowel, omentum and other organs, which increases the risk of injury (Figs. 6.1, 6.2, 6.3, 6.4, and 6.5) (Table 6.8).

Perspective

Incisional hernias can be asymptomatic, but many cause discomfort rather than bowel obstruction. Because of the narrow defect in some cases, chronic incarceration of pre-peritoneal fat is not uncommon, and these herniae may be irreducible. The risk of infection is increased when bowel is obstructed. If bowel obstruction is present, the offending loop must be visualized and its viability assessed at the time of repair. This may require extension of the incision or conversion to full laparotomy to assess bowel viability. The usual complications associated with abdominal wall surgery are seen. Monofilament, nonabsorbable suture is usually used to repair the defect. Plastic mesh is sometimes used; however, this slightly increases the risk of foreign body reactions and infection. Closure of the abdominal wall is associated with a real—probably truly unknown—incidence of wound failure that eventually leads to incisional herniation. The development of a wound herniation may be overt or go unrecognized for many years. Later development is also recognized. Although often difficult to assess the etiology of an incisional hernia, wound failure is most commonly related to infection and infectious wound complications, but may be related to the actual surgical closure technique. The incidence of failure of wound healing and incisional hernias can be decreased by certain closure techniques, but some will still develop. Many hernias remain asymptomatic. Symptomatic incisional hernias, with intermittent pain, incarceration and obstruction are well recognized. The symptoms vary from vague abdominal pain to full-blown bowel obstruction and repair is indicated. Recurrence rates are difficult to formally assess in prospective trials, but are generally considered to be frequent. A key element in the repair of any incisional hernia is exploration of the entire wound for evidence of defects; clinically, with ultrasound imaging, or intra-operatively by digital palpation or direct visualization inside the abdominal wall, thus avoiding missing of a defect that is present and not previously evident. Failure to explore the entire wound leads in part to the high "recurrence" rate. It is not necessarily a recurrence, simply

Fig. 6.1 Extruding infected inguinal hernia mesh

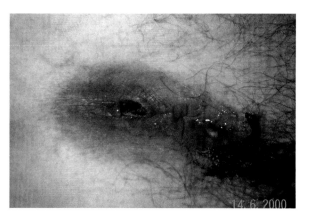

Fig. 6.2 Another image of extruding infected inguinal hernia mesh

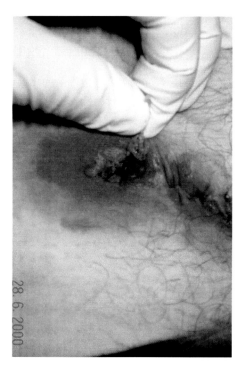

a missed defect that requires re-operation. Wounds generally do not fail in any one specific area; the entire wound is at risk for failure at any time. Seroma and hematoma are well-recognized complications of any ventral hernia repair, likely related to the wider dissection needed to accomplish the repair. They are more frequent in the repair of these hernias than in the repair of the more common groin herniae. These can generally be managed conservatively or by frequent needle aspirations. Bowel injury during the repair is possible at any time. The use of mesh is associated

Fig. 6.3 Removed infected
inguinal hernia mesh

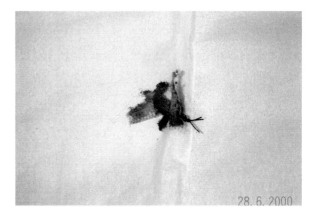

Fig. 6.4 Infected inguinal
hernia repair

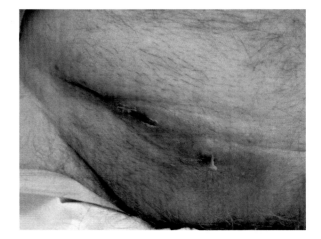

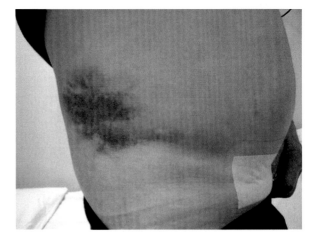

Fig. 6.5 Hernia hematoma

Table 6.8 Surgery for small incisional hernia estimated frequency of complications, risks, and consequences

Complications, risks, and consequences	Estimated frequency
Most significant/serious complications	
Bleeding or hematoma formation[a]	5–20 %
Infection[a]	0.1–1 %
Urinary retention	1–5 %
Hernia recurrence[a] (10 year)	5–20 %
Rare significant/serious problems	
Vascular injury—artery or vein[a]	0.1–1[a] %
Laparotomy (bowel injury or adhesion related strangulation or ischemia)[a]	0.1–1 %
Small bowel obstruction[a]	0.1–1 %
Deep venous thrombosis[a]	0.1–1 %
Dehiscence[a]	<0.1 %
Less serious complications	
Pain/discomfort/tenderness (wound)[a]	
Acute (<4 weeks)	20–50 %
Chronic (>12 weeks)	0.1–1 %
Numbness/altered sensation	0.1–1[a] %
Bruising	50–80 %
Seroma formation	5–20 %
Local swelling	20–50 %
Suture abscess/granuloma formation ± suture sinus[a]	0.1–1 %
Wound scarring	1–5 %
Dimpling/deformity of the skin[a]	1–5 %
Drain tube(s)[a]	1–5 %

[a]Dependent on underlying pathology, anatomy, surgical technique, and preferences

with bowel complications to some extent and some surgeons prefer not to place mesh directly against the bowel, if possible. Peritoneum can be placed above the mesh to perhaps minimize mesh-bowel related complications. Because the contents of the hernia sac are often difficult to appreciate (even with imaging) in the preoperative evaluation, injury to the bowel is more likely in the repair of incisional hernias.

Major Complications

Infections are mainly of skin (*S. aureus*) origin; however, bowel derived organisms (*E. coli*; bacteroides sp.; Strep pyogenes) may be causative when bowel is obstructed or breached. Infection often necessitates removal of some or all foreign material such as sutures and mesh and may dictate later hernia repair. Infection also increases the risk of suture sinus, **dehiscence**, and hernia recurrence. **Bleeding** may occur from vessels associated with the edge of the peritoneal hernial sac, and especially from omental vessels that are often thin walled and easily traumatized. Occasionally mesenteric vessels can be traumatized during reduction of bowel causing bleeding.

These situations do not usually present difficulty in obtaining control of bleeding. **Bowel injury** is a potentially serious problem and can occur easily if ischemia and/ or infarction of bowel is present. Extension of the incision or midline conventional **laparotomy** is often safest to fully inspect the bowel. Occasionally perforation has occurred and infection is established before surgery. This can present some difficulty with regard to repair using a nonabsorbable suture or mesh. However, mass closure using monofilament sutures is usually satisfactory. Avoidance of mesh, or any foreign material that is more than absolutely necessary for closure, is advisable. Rarely, delayed primary closure is indicated, with subsequent delayed elective hernia repair some months later. **Suture sinus** may develop as a result of a foreign body reaction to suture material, especially knots, or mesh. Infection can cause or be secondary to suture sinuses. When established, a suture sinus will usually only settle after removal of the offending foreign material. However, removal of some of the material may be sufficient, and then the main bulk of material used in the repair can be retained. Sometimes, however, all foreign material has to be removed to heal the sinus and/or infection. There is a recognized greater incidence of **hernia recurrence** after incisional hernia repair, and patients should be warned about this; however, in the majority of cases it is usually not problematic. **Seroma formation** produces a lump which usually settles and may need regular needle aspiration drainage(s) to assist this.

Consent and Risk Reduction

Main Points to Explain

- Discomfort
- Bleeding
- Infection
- Bowel perforation
- Recurrent hernia
- Laparotomy
- Further surgery
- Risks without surgery

Surgery for Large Incisional Hernia

Description

General anesthesia is usually used; however, local infiltration and occasionally high spinal anesthesia can be used in highly selected cases, with or without neuroleptic agents. Incisional hernia is a relatively common surgical problem. It typically occurs through a defect in a previous scar allowing abdominal contents to protrude, sometimes containing peritoneum and shows as a bulge, emphasized by coughing. The contents are often pre-peritoneal fat, occasionally omentum and less commonly bowel within a peritoneal sac. It is observed in all ages and both genders almost equally. In obese patients the diagnosis may be especially difficult. Elective repair is indicated in symptomatic patients; incarceration and bowel obstruction require emergency intervention. Non-operative reduction may be useful to reduce urgency if the period of irreducibility is less than 4 or so hours, depending on the degree of ischemia. Incision/excision of the previous scar is usually appropriate for access; however, a separate longitudinal midline or transverse skin incision may be used. The sac is defined and excised at the edge of the defect to expose the contents before reduction. An incision through the edge of the defect may be used if better access is needed to reduce or inspect the hernial contents. Not infrequently the hernia is multi-loculated, necessitating more dissection which usually increases the risk of complications (Figs. 6.6, 6.7, 6.8, 6.9, and 6.10).

Fig. 6.6 Infected abdominal incisional hernia mesh

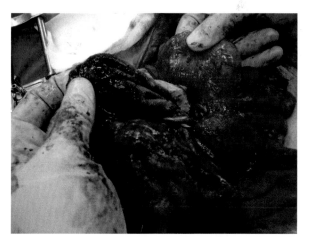

Fig. 6.7 Infected abdominal incisional hernia mesh removed

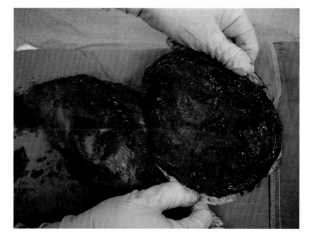

Fig. 6.8 Vacuum dressing
in place

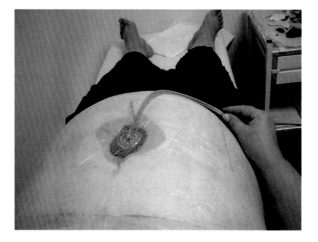

Fig. 6.9 Healing wound after
vacuum dressing

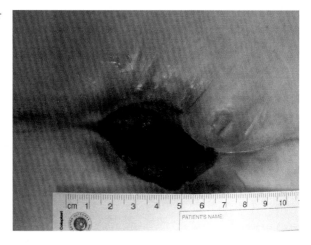

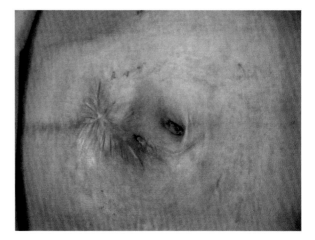

Fig. 6.10 Wound sinus
infected mesh

Anatomical Points

The anatomy of the region of the previous incision and the contents usually determine the nature, surgical difficulty, and risk of complications. Divarication of the rectus muscles may produce a broad bulge especially evident on lifting the head from the lying position, potentially appearing similar to a midline incisional hernia. In the relaxed recumbent patient an incisional hernia can often be gently inverted to palpate a distinct edge to the defect, and sometimes, abdominal contents. It protrudes on coughing (especially when standing), exhibiting a "cough impulse," whereas in divarication the abdominal wall tends to tighten and any "cough impulse" is much less, or absent. Occasionally an incisional hernia is irreducible and a mass is palpable often with a narrow (constricting) neck. The hernia may protrude through all layers of the abdominal wall, producing the "classical" signs of an incisional hernia. Not infrequently the incisional hernia lies between musculo-fascial layers, where the signs may be less prominent, and the hernia not as easily palpated. At operation the sac and edge of the defect must be anatomically dissected and defined. Multiple hernial openings are not infrequent making the sac irregular in shape, with adhesions tethering bowel, omentum and other organs, which increases the risk of injury. In massive herniae, pneumo-peritoneum may be induced for some weeks preoperatively to expand the abdomen and allow for respiratory adjustment to cope with the return of the large hernial contents to the abdomen (Table 6.9).

Table 6.9 Surgery for large incisional hernia estimated frequency of complications, risks, and consequences

Complications, risks, and consequences	Estimated frequency
Most significant/serious complications	
Bleeding or hematoma formation[a]	5–20 %
Infection[a]	1–5 %
Neural injury[a]—iliohypogastric, subcostal, etc.	1–5 %
Vascular injury—mesenteric, omental artery or vein[a]	1–5 %
Hernia recurrence[a] (10 year)	5–20 %
Small bowel obstruction[a]	1–5 %
Urinary retention	1–5 %
Rare significant/serious problems	
Laparotomy (bowel injury or adhesion related strangulation or ischemia)[a]	0.1–1 %
Skin ulceration[a]	0.1–1 %
Colostomy or ileostomy[a]	0.1–1 %
Deep venous thrombosis[a]	0.1–1 %
Dehiscence	<0.1 %
Mortality[a,b] (overall)	<0.1 %
Less serious complications	
Pain/discomfort/tenderness (wound/testicular/thigh pain)[a]	
Acute (<4 weeks)	20–50 %
Chronic (>12 weeks)	0.1–1 %

(continued)

Table 6.9 (continued)

Complications, risks, and consequences	Estimated frequency
Numbness/altered sensation	0.1–1[a] %
Bruising	50–80 %
Seroma formation	5–20 %
Local swelling	20–50 %
Suture abscess/granuloma formation ± suture sinus[a]	0.1–1 %
Wound scarring	1–5 %
Dimpling/deformity of the skin[a]	1–5 %
Drain tube(s)[a]	1–5 %

[a]Dependent on underlying pathology, anatomy, surgical technique, and preferences
[b]Mortality may be higher in some settings related to individual patient comorbidities

Perspective

Large incisional herniae can be asymptomatic, but many cause discomfort rather than bowel obstruction. Discomfort due to mesenteric "traction" is not uncommon. Most of the discussion for small incisional herniae applies more so to larger herniae. Because of the narrow defect in some cases, chronic incarceration with abdominal contents, often bowel, is not uncommon, and these herniae may be irreducible. The risk of infection is increased when bowel is obstructed. If bowel obstruction is present, the offending loop must be visualized and its viability assessed at the time of repair. This may require extension of the incision or conversion to full laparotomy to assess bowel viability. The usual complications associated with abdominal wall surgery are seen. Massive incisional hernias of the abdominal wall can present a particularly unique challenge to the surgeon. Composite techniques or prosthetics with or without rotation of tissue flaps adds complexity to the procedure and additional risk of wound complications. Repair often entails wide dissection of the abdominal wall with an increased opportunity for hematoma and seroma formation and loss of tissue. While the objective is to attain closure of the fascia with tissue, it is not always possible without creating intra-abdominal tension with its associated pulmonary and cardiovascular effects. Ideally mesh or other material should be placed in the pre-peritoneal space, below the anterior rectus fascia and above the peritoneum to minimize adhesions to the bowel which can engender complications of significant magnitude. Placement of the mesh as an "on-lay patch" to the rectus fascia has an increased incidence of failure compared to mesh placed below the fascia. Suture granulomas and injury to peripheral and intercostal nerves is related to the placement of mesh below the fascia and the use of large "through and through" sutures to secure it. The bowel is at risk of injury, which can lead to peritonitis which can be fatal. Serotomies not noted at repair of an incisional hernia can evolve in a short period of time to full thickness bowel wall necrosis and fistula formation or peritonitis. The bowel is especially at risk during repair of a recurrent incisional hernia because of the scarring and distortion of normal anatomy. Suture complications are more related to the material used and the presence of infection than the actual placement. The use of nonabsorbable monofilament suture has minimized suture-related complications and its use is encouraged to avoid the granulomas and infections seen in years past. The laparoscopic approach to the repair of incisional hernias has been gaining momentum in recent years. While the concept has appeal, the complications associated with access to an abdomen with adhesions are increased. Specifically, an increased incidence of enterotomy associated with either the access or the dissection is especially problematic given the mandatory use of a prosthetic material. Recurrence rates are difficult to formally assess in prospective trials, but are generally considered to be more frequent than for any other type of hernia. However, weaker tissues and failure to explore the entire wound leads in part to the high "recurrence" (missed defect) rate. Mesh is usually used and therefore mesh-related complications are more common. Because the contents of the hernia sac are often multi-loculated and more difficult to appreciate in the intra-operative evaluation (even on imaging), injury to the bowel is more likely in the repair of larger incisional hernias.

Major Complications

Infections are mainly of skin (*S. aureus*) origin; however, bowel derived organisms (*E. coli*; bacteroides sp.; Strep pyogenes) may be causative when bowel is obstructed or breached. Infection often necessitates removal of some or all foreign material such as sutures and mesh and may dictate later hernia repair. Infection also increases the risk of suture sinus, **dehiscence**, and hernia recurrence. **Bleeding** may occur from vessels associated with the edge of the peritoneal hernial sac, and especially from omental vessels that are often thin walled and easily traumatized. Occasionally mesenteric vessels can be traumatized during reduction of bowel causing bleeding. These situations do not usually present difficulty in obtaining control of bleeding. **Bowel injury** is a potentially serious problem and can occur easily if ischemia and/or infarction of bowel is present. Extension of the incision or midline conventional **laparotomy** is often safest to fully inspect the bowel. Occasionally perforation has occurred and infection is established before surgery. This can present some difficulty with regard to repair using a nonabsorbable suture or mesh. However, mass closure using monofilament sutures is usually satisfactory. Avoidance of mesh, or any foreign material than is more than absolutely necessary for closure, is advisable. Rarely, delayed primary closure is indicated, with subsequent delayed elective hernia repair some months later. Very rarely, **colostomy or ileostomy** may be required following bowel injury and patients should usually be warned of this small possibility. **Skin ulceration** is occasionally seen with massive herniae, often due to abrasion. **Suture sinus** may develop as a result of a foreign body reaction to suture material, especially knots, or mesh. Infection can cause or be secondary to suture sinuses. When established, a suture sinus will usually only settle after removal of the offending foreign material. However, removal of some of the material may be sufficient, and then the main bulk of material used in the repair can be retained. Sometimes, however, all foreign material has to be removed to heal the sinus and/or infection. There is a recognized higher incidence of **hernia recurrence** after large incisional hernia repair, and patients should be warned about this; however, in the majority of cases it is usually not problematic. **Seroma formation** produces a lump which usually settles and may need regular needle aspiration drainage(s) to assist this.

Consent and Risk Reduction

Main Points to Explain

- Discomfort
- Bleeding
- Infection
- Bowel perforation
- Recurrent hernia
- Laparotomy
- Further surgery
- Risks without surgery

Surgery for Para-Stomal Hernia

Description

General anesthesia is usually used; however, local infiltration and occasionally high spinal anesthesia can be used in highly selected cases, with or without systemic neuroleptic agents. Para-stomal hernia is a relatively common surgical problem. It typically occurs through a defect at the edge of a stomal opening for an ileostomy or colostomy, allowing abdominal contents to protrude, covered by peritoneum and shows as a bulge, emphasized by coughing at the side of the stoma. It may deform the stoma and bag. The contents are often pre-peritoneal fat, occasionally omentum and less commonly bowel within a peritoneal sac. It is observed in all ages and both genders almost equally. In obese patients, the diagnosis may be especially difficult. Elective repair is indicated in symptomatic patients; incarceration and bowel obstruction require emergency intervention. Non-operative reduction may be useful to reduce urgency if the period of irreducibility is less than 4 or so hours, depending on the degree of ischemia. Incision/excision of the previous scar is usually appropriate for access; however, a separate longitudinal midline or transverse skin incision may be used. The sac is defined and excised at the edge of the defect to expose the contents before reduction. An incision through the edge of the defect may be used if better access is needed to reduce or inspect the hernial contents. Not infrequently, the hernia is multi-loculated, necessitating more dissection, which usually increases the risk of complications.

Anatomical Points

The anatomy of the region of the previous incision and stoma usually determines the contents, nature, and risk of complications. In the relaxed recumbent patient a para-stomal hernia can often be gently inverted to palpate a distinct edge to the defect, and sometimes, abdominal contents. It protrudes on coughing (especially when standing), exhibiting a "cough impulse." Occasionally, a para-stomal hernia is irreducible and a mass is palpable often with a narrow (constricting) neck. The hernia may protrude through all layers of the abdominal wall, producing the "classical" signs of an incisional hernia. Not infrequently the hernia lies between musculo-fascial layers, where the signs may be less prominent, and the hernia not as easily palpated. At operation the sac and edge of the defect must be anatomically dissected and defined. Multiple hernial openings or loculations can occur making the sac irregular in shape, with adhesions tethering bowel, omentum, and other organs, which increases the risk of injury (Table 6.10).

Table 6.10 Surgery for para-stomal hernia estimated frequency of complications, risks, and consequences

Complications, risks, and consequences	Estimated frequency
Most significant/serious complications	
Bleeding or hematoma formation[a]	5–20 %
Infection[a]	1–5 %
Vascular injury—mesenteric, omental artery or vein[a]	1–5 %
Urinary retention	1–5 %
Small bowel obstruction[a]	1–5 %
Hernia recurrence[a] (10 year)	5–20 %
Rare significant/serious problems	
Full laparotomy (bowel injury or adhesion related strangulation or ischemia)[a]	0.1–1 %
Revision of colostomy or ileostomy[a]	0.1–1 %
Dehiscence	<0.1 %
Mortality[a]	<0.1 %
Less serious complications	
Pain/discomfort/tenderness (wound/testicular/thigh pain)[a]	
Acute (<4 weeks)	20–50 %
Chronic (>12 weeks)	0.1–1 %
Numbness/altered sensation	0.1–1[a] %
Bruising	50–80 %
Seroma formation	5–20 %
Local swelling	20–50 %
Suture abscess/granuloma formation ± suture sinus[a]	0.1–1 %
Wound scarring	1–5 %
Dimpling/deformity of the skin[a]	1–5 %
Drain tube(s)[a]	1–5 %

[a]Dependent on underlying pathology, anatomy, surgical technique, and preferences

Perspective

Para-stomal herniae can be asymptomatic, but many cause discomfort or poor adherence of the stomal bag, rather than bowel obstruction. Because of the narrow defect in some cases, chronic incarceration with abdominal contents, often bowel, is not uncommon, and these herniae may be irreducible. The risk of infection is increased when bowel is obstructed or densely adherent. If bowel obstruction is present, the offending loop must be visualized and its viability assessed at the time of repair. This may require extension of the incision or conversion to full laparotomy to assess bowel viability. The usual complications associated with abdominal wall surgery are seen. Massive hernias of the abdominal wall can present a particularly unique challenge to the surgeon. Composite techniques or prosthetics with or without rotation of tissue flaps adds complexity to the procedure and additional risk of wound complications. Repair often entails wide dissection of the abdominal wall with an increased opportunity for hematoma and seroma formation and loss of tissue. While the objective is to attain closure of the fascia with tissue, it is not always possible without creating intra-abdominal tension with its associated pulmonary and cardiovascular effects. Ideally mesh or other material should be avoided, or if necessary placed on the anterior abdominal wall or in the pre-peritoneal space, below the anterior rectus fascia and above the peritoneum to minimize adhesions to the bowel which can engender complications of significant magnitude. Suture granulomas and injury to peripheral and intercostal nerves are related to the placement of mesh below the fascia and the use of large 'through and through' sutures to secure it. The bowel is at risk of injury, which can lead to peritonitis, which can be fatal. Serotomies not noted at repair can evolve in a short period of time to full thickness bowel wall necrosis and fistula formation or peritonitis. The bowel is especially at risk during repair of recurrent para-stomal hernias, because of the scarring and distortion of normal anatomy. Suture complications are more related to the material used and the presence of infection than the actual placement. The use of nonabsorbable monofilament suture has minimized suture-related complications and its use is encouraged to avoid the granulomas and infections seen in years past. Recurrence rates are difficult to formally assess in prospective trials, but are generally considered to be more frequent than for most other types of hernia. However, weaker tissues and failure to explore the entire wound lead in part to the high "recurrence" (missed defect) rate. Because the contents of the hernia sac may be adherent and multi-loculated, they are more difficult to appreciate in the intra-operative evaluation, injury to the bowel is more likely in the repair of these hernias.

Major Complications

Infections are mainly of skin (*S. aureus*) origin; however, bowel derived organisms (*E. coli*; bacteroides sp.; Strep pyogenes) may be causative when bowel is obstructed or breached. Infection often necessitates removal of some or all foreign material such as sutures and mesh and may dictate later hernia repair. Infection also increases the risk of suture sinus, dehiscence, and hernia recurrence. **Bleeding** may occur from vessels associated with the edge of the peritoneal hernial sac, and especially from omental vessels that are often thin walled and easily traumatized. Occasionally mesenteric vessels can be traumatized during reduction of bowel causing bleeding. These situations do not usually present difficulty in obtaining control of bleeding. **Bowel injury** is a potentially serious problem and can occur easily if ischemia and/or infarction of bowel is present. Extension of the incision or midline conventional **laparotomy** is often safest to fully inspect the bowel, if required. Occasionally, **perforation** has occurred and infection is established before surgery. This can present some difficulty with regard to repair using a non-absorbable suture or mesh. However, mass closure using monofilament sutures is usually satisfactory. Avoidance of mesh, or any foreign material that is more than absolutely necessary for closure, is advisable. Rarely, delayed primary closure is indicated, with subsequent delayed elective hernia repair some months later. Very rarely, **colostomy or ileostomy revision** may be required following bowel injury and patients should usually be warned of this small possibility. **Suture sinus** may develop as a result of a foreign body reaction to suture material, especially knots, or mesh. Infection can cause or be secondary to suture sinuses. When established, a suture sinus will usually only settle after removal of the offending foreign material. However, removal of some of the material may be sufficient, and then the main bulk of material used in the repair can be retained. Sometimes, however, all foreign material has to be removed to heal the sinus and/or infection. There is a recognized higher incidence of **hernia recurrence** after para-stomal hernia repair, and patients should be warned about this; however, in the majority of cases it is usually not problematic. **Seroma formation** produces a lump, which usually settles and may need **needle aspiration drainage(s)** to assist this. **Multi-system organ failure** and **mortality** are rare, but are reported after **peritonitis and systemic sepsis**, and/or cardiovascular events.

Consent and Risk Reduction

Main Points to Explain

- Discomfort
- Bleeding
- Infection
- Bowel perforation
- Recurrent hernia
- Laparotomy
- Stomal dysfunction
- Further surgery
- Risks without surgery

Acknowledgments The authors would like to thank and acknowledge the following experienced clinician who discussed the chapters and acted as an advisor, Professor Jonathan Meakins, Monteal, Canada and Oxford, UK.

Further Reading, References, and Resources

Surgery for Epigastric Hernia

Bennett D. Incidence and management of primary abdominal wall hernias: umbilical, epigastric and spigelian. In: Fitzgibbons RJ, Greenburg AG, editors. Nyhus and Condon's hernia. 5th ed. Philadelphia: Lippincott Williams and Wilkins; 2002. p. 389–414.

Hugh TB, Chen FC, Hugh TJ. Divarication of the recti, or abdominal incisional hernia? A simple differentiating clinical test. ANZ J Surg. 1991;61:819–20.

Surgery for Umbilical/Paraumbilical Hernia

Bennett D. Incidence and management of primary abdominal wall hernias: umbilical, epigastric and spigelian. In: Fitzgibbons RJ, Greenburg AG, editors. Nyhus and Condon's hernia. 5th ed. Philadelphia: Lippincott Williams and Wilkins; 2002. p. 389–414.

Surgery for Primary Open Inguinal Hernia

Amid PK, Shulman AG, Lichtenstein IL. Open. "tension-free" repair of inguinal hernias: the Lichtenstein technique. Eur J Surg. 1996;162:447–53.

Bay-Nielsen M, Perkins FM, Kehlet H. Pain and functional impairment 1 year after inguinal herniorrhaphy: a nationwide questionnaire study. Ann Surg. 2001;233:1–7.

Bringman S, Blomqvist P. Intestinal obstruction after inguinal and femoral hernia repair: a study of 33,275 operations during 1992–2000 in Sweden. Hernia. 2005;9(2):178–83.

Bringman S, Ramel S, Heikkinen TJ, Englund T, Westman B, Anderberg B. Tension-free inguinal hernia repair: TEP versus mesh-plug versus Lichtenstein: a prospective randomized controlled trial. Ann Surg. 2003;237(1):142–7.

Cassar K, Munro A. Surgical treatment of incisional hernia. Br J Surg. 2002;89(5):534–45.

Clemente CD. Anatomy – a regional atlas of the human body. 4th ed. Baltimore: Williams and Wilkins; 1997.

Collaboration EH. Mesh compared with non-mesh methods of open groin hernia repair: systematic review of randomized controlled trials. Br J Surg. 2000;87:854–9.

den Hartog D, Dur AH, Tuinebreijer WE, Kreis RW. Open surgical procedures for incisional hernias. Cochrane Database Syst Rev. 2008;(3):CD006438.

European Union Hernia Trialists Collaboration. Mesh compared to non-mesh methods of open groin hernia repair: systematic review of randomized controlled trials. Br J Surg. 2000; 87:854–9.

Geis WP, Singh K, Gillian GK. An algorithm for the treatment of chronic groin pain after inguinal herniorraphy. In: Fitzgibbons RJ, Greenburg AG, editors. Nyhus and Condon's hernia. 5th ed. Philadelphia: Lippincott Williams and Wilkins; 2002. p. 305–16.

Greenburg AG. Revisiting the recurrent groin hernia. Am J Surg. 1987;154:34–40.

Healy M, Shackford SR, Osler TM, et al. Complications in surgical patients. Arch Surg. 2002;137:611–618.

Jamieson GG. The anatomy of general surgical operations. 2nd ed. Edinburgh: Churchill Livingston; 2006.

Kugel RD. Minimally invasive, nonlaparoscopic, preperitoneal, and sutureless, inguinal herniorrhaphy. Am J Surg. 1999;178:298–302.

Nilsson E, Kald A, Anderberg B, et al. Hernia surgery in a defined population: a prospective three-year audit. Eur J Surg. 1997;163:823–9.

Rutkow IM. Surgical operations in the United States. Then (1983) and now (1994). Arch Surg. 1997;132:983–90.

Rutkow IM, Robbins AW. "Tension-free" inguinal herniorrhaphy: a preliminary report on the "mesh plug" technique. Surgery. 1993;114:3–8.

Scott NW, McCormack K, Graham P, Go PM, Ross SJ, Grant AM. Open mesh versus non-mesh for repair of femoral and inguinal hernia. Cochrane Database Syst Rev. 2002;(4):CD002197.

Surgery for Recurrent Open Inguinal Hernia

Clemente CD. Anatomy – a regional atlas of the human body. 4th ed. Baltimore: Williams and Wilkins; 1997.

Greenburg AG. Revisiting the recurrent groin hernia. Am J Surg. 1987;154(1):35–40.

Haapaniemi S, Gunnarsson U, Nordin P, Nilsson E. Reoperation after recurrent groin hernia repair. Ann Surg. 2001;234(1):122–6.

Jamieson GG. The anatomy of general surgical operations. 2nd ed. Edinburgh: Churchill Livingston; 2006.

Sevonius D, Gunnarsson U, Nordin P, Nilsson E, Sandblom G. Repeated groin hernia recurrences. Ann Surg. 2009;249(3):516–8.

Surgery for Laparoscopic (Pre-Peritoneal Approach)

Clemente CD. Anatomy – a regional atlas of the human body. 4th ed. Baltimore: Williams and Wilkins; 1997.

Crawford DL, Phillips EH. Laparoscopic totally extraperitoneal herniorrhaphy. In: Fitzgibbons RJ, Greenburg AG, editors. Nyhus and Condon's hernia. 5th ed. Philadelphia: Lippincott Williams and Wilkins; 2002. p. 238–53.

Jamieson GG. The anatomy of general surgical operations. 2nd ed. Edinburgh: Churchill Livingston; 2006.

Papadakis K, Greenburg AG. Preperitoneal hernia repair. In: Fitzgibbons RJ, Greenburg AG, editors. Nyhus and Condon's hernia. 5th ed. Philadelphia: Lippincott Williams and Wilkins; 2002. p. 181–98.

Surgery for Laparoscopic (Intra/Trans-Peritoneal Approach)

Clemente CD. Anatomy – a regional atlas of the human body. 4th ed. Baltimore: Williams and Wilkins; 1997.

Fitzgibbons RJ, Filipi CJ. The transabdominal preperitoneal laparoscopic herniorrhaphy. In: Fitzgibbons RJ, Greenburg AG, editors. Nyhus and Condon's hernia. 5th ed. Philadelphia: Lippincott Williams and Wilkins; 2002. p. 255–68.

Jamieson GG. The anatomy of general surgical operations. 2nd ed. Edinburgh: Churchill Livingston; 2006.

Ridings P, Evans DS. The transabdominal pre-peritoneal (TAPP) inguinal hernia repair: a trip along the learning curve. J R Coll Surg Edinb. 2000;45(2):29–32.

Wake BL, McCormack K, Fraser C, Vale L, Perez J, Grant A. Transabdominal pre-peritoneal (TAPP) vs totally extraperitoneal (TEP) laparoscopic techniques for inguinal hernia repair. Cochrane Database Syst Rev. 2005;(1). Art. No.:CD004703. doi:10.1002/14651858. CD004703.pub2.

Surgery for Femoral Hernia Repair

Clemente CD. Anatomy – a regional atlas of the human body. 4th ed. Baltimore: Williams and Wilkins; 1997.

Jamieson GG. The anatomy of general surgical operations. 2nd ed. Edinburgh: Churchill Livingston; 2006.

Surgery for Small Incisional Hernia

Bennett D. Incidence and management of primary abdominal wall hernias: umbilical, epigastric and spigelian. In: Fitzgibbons RJ, Greenburg AG, editors. Nyhus and Condon's hernia. 5th ed. Philadelphia: Lippincott Williams and Wilkins; 2002. p. 389–414.

Clemente CD. Anatomy – a regional atlas of the human body. 4th ed. Baltimore: Williams and Wilkins; 1997.

Hugh TB, Chen FC, Hugh TJ. Divarication of the recti, or abdominal incisional hernia? A simple differentiating clinical test. ANZ J Surg. 1991;61:819–20.

Jamieson GG. The anatomy of general surgical operations. 2nd ed. Edinburgh: Churchill Livingston; 2006.

Surgery for Large Incisional Hernia

Bennett D. Incidence and management of primary abdominal wall hernias: umbilical, epigastric and spigelian. In: Fitzgibbons RJ, Greenburg AG, editors. Nyhus and Condon's hernia. 5th ed. Philadelphia: Lippincott Williams and Wilkins; 2002. p. 389–414.

Clemente CD. Anatomy – a regional atlas of the human body. 4th ed. Baltimore: Williams and Wilkins; 1997.

Hugh TB, Chen FC, Hugh TJ. Divarication of the recti, or abdominal incisional hernia? A simple differentiating clinical test. ANZ J Surg. 1991;61:819–20.

Jamieson GG. The anatomy of general surgical operations. 2nd ed. Edinburgh: Churchill Livingston; 2006.

Surgery for Parastomal Hernia

Aldridge AJ, Simson JN. Erosion and perforation of colon by synthetic mesh in a recurrent para-colostomy hernia. Hernia. 2001;5(2):110–2.

Amin SN, Armitage NC, Abercrombie JF, Scholefield JH. Lateral repair of parastomal hernia. Ann R Coll Surg Engl. 2001;83(3):206–8.

Baig MK, Larach JA, Chang S, Long C, Weiss EG, Nogueras JJ, Wexner SD. Outcome of parastomal hernia repair with and without midline laparotomy. Tech Coloproctol. 2006;10(4):282–6.

Clemente CD. Anatomy – a regional atlas of the human body. 4th ed. Baltimore: Williams and Wilkins; 1997.

Craft RO, Huguet KL, McLemore EC, Harold KL. Laparoscopic parastomal hernia repair. Hernia. 2008;12(2):137–40.

Franklin Jr ME, Treviño JM, Portillo G, Vela I, Glass JL, González JJ. The use of porcine small intestinal submucosa as a prosthetic material for laparoscopic hernia repair in infected and potentially contaminated fields: long-term follow-up. Surg Endosc. 2008;22(9):1941–6.

Geisler DJ, Reilly JC, Vaughan SG, Glennon EJ, Kondylis PD. Safety and outcome of use of nonabsorbable mesh for repair of fascial defects in the presence of open bowel. Dis Colon Rectum. 2003;46(8):1118–23.

Hogg ME, King PM, Keenan RA. A modified lateral approach to parastomal hernia repair. Surgeon. 2009;7(1):56–8.

Jamieson GG. The anatomy of general surgical operations. 2nd ed. Edinburgh: Churchill Livingston; 2006.

Kelly ME, Behrman SW. The safety and efficacy of prosthetic hernia repair in clean-contaminated and contaminated wounds. Am Surg. 2002;68(6):524–8. discussion 528–9.

Lüning TH, Spillenaar-Bilgen EJ. Parastomal hernia: complications of extra-peritoneal onlay mesh placement. Hernia. 2009;13(5):487–90.

McGreevy JM, Goodney PP, Birkmeyer CM, Finlayson SR, Laycock WS, Birkmeyer JD. A prospective study comparing the complication rates between laparoscopic and open ventral hernia repairs. Surg Endosc. 2003;17(11):1778–80.

McLemore EC, Harold KL, Efron JE, Laxa BU, Young-Fadok TM, Heppell JP. Parastomal hernia: short-term outcome after laparoscopic and conventional repairs. Surg Innov. 2007;14(3):199–204.

Rieger N, Moore J, Hewett P, Lee S, Stephens J. Parastomal hernia repair. Colorectal Dis. 2004;6(3):203–5.

Saclarides TJ, Hsu A, Quiros R. In situ mesh repair of parastomal hernias. Am Surg. 2004;70(8):701–5.

Steele SR, Lee P, Martin MJ, Mullenix PS, Sullivan ES. Is parastomal hernia repair with polypropylene mesh safe? Am J Surg. 2003;185(5):436–40.

Chapter 7
Head and Neck Surgery

Brendon J. Coventry, Guy Rees, and Christopher O'Brien[†]

General Perspective and Overview

The relative risks and complications increase proportionately according to the nature, site of the mass or problem, extent of procedure performed, technique, or complexity of the problem. Large masses, inflammatory masses, and those of malignant etiology often carry higher risks of bleeding and infection than smaller ones, in general terms. Similarly, risk is relatively higher for recurrent and complex surgery, and for those closer to neural structures (e.g., facial or laryngeal nerves).

Knowledge of the anatomy and the variations commonly seen is helpful in minimizing nerve and vessel injury. Surgeons argue the benefits of one approach over the other, but there is little data to demonstrate differences in terms of the observed or reported complications. Other surgeons will argue that the use of drains adds to the complication rates, but that is perhaps less of a consideration in the current era. Tracheostomy procedures are aimed at provision of a semi-permanent airway, and as such, may be urgent emergency operations, or elective, and carry the risk of

[†]Deceased

B.J. Coventry, BMBS, PhD, FRACS, FACS, FRSM (✉)
Discipline of Surgery, Royal Adelaide Hospital, University of Adelaide,
L5 Eleanor Harrald Building, North Terrace, 5000 Adelaide, SA, Australia
e-mail: brendon.coventry@adelaide.edu.au

G. Rees, MBBS, FRACS
Department of Ear, Nose and Throat Surgery,
Royal Adelaide Hospital, University of Adelaide,
L5 Eleanor Harrald Building, North Terrace, 5000 Adelaide, SA, Australia

C. O'Brien[†], MS, MD, FRCS (HON), FRACS
Sydney Head and Neck Cancer Institute, Sydney, NSW, Australia

B.J. Coventry (ed.), *Peripheral, Head and Neck Surgery*,
Surgery: Complications, Risks and Consequences,
DOI 10.1007/978-1-4471-5415-0_7, © Springer-Verlag London 2014

airway obstruction and oxygen desaturation, which is usually greater in the emergency setting.

Possible reduction in the risk of misunderstandings over complications or consequences from head and neck surgery might be achieved by:

- Good explanation of the risks, aims, benefits, and limitations of the procedure(s)
- Useful planning considering the anatomy, approach, alternatives, and method
- Avoiding likely associated vessels and nerves
- Adequate clinical follow-up

With these factors and facts in mind, the information given in this chapter must be appropriately and discernibly interpreted and used.

IMPORTANT NOTE: It should be emphasized that the risks and frequencies that are given here *represent derived figures*. These *figures are best estimates of relative frequencies across most institutions*, not merely the highest-performing ones, and as such are often representative of a number of studies, which include different patients with differing comorbidities and different surgeons. In addition, the risks of complications in lower or higher risk patients may lie outside these estimated ranges, and individual clinical judgement is required as to the expected risks communicated to the patient, staff, or for other purposes. The range of risks is also derived from experience and the literature; while risks outside this range may exist, certain risks may be reduced or absent due to variations of procedures or surgical approaches. It is recognized that different patients, practitioners, institutions, regions, and countries may vary in their requirements and recommendations.

The risks of combined or associated surgery need to be considered and usually added to those risks determined below, where procedures are performed together.

For lymph node surgery or for thyroid/parathyroid surgery, please (see Volume 3), or for other biopsies used to obtain diagnosis, please refer to Volume 2.

Percutaneous Mini-Tracheostomy

Description

Local anesthesia is used, typically in the sedated, unconscious, or anesthetized ICU patient. The percutaneous needle approach is usually less traumatic than the open approach and is being used by ICU clinicians more widely because of the relative ease and convenience. It requires little surgical experience, but anatomical knowledge is still essential. The Seldinger type approach is the most commonly used internationally. The trachea is palpated (ultrasound may be used, particularly if edema is present or the anatomy is otherwise obscured), the patient is pre-oxygenated, the endotracheal tube is retracted to just below the glottis, and a large-bore needle is placed directly into the trachea angled slightly inferiorly. A guidewire is placed through this and threaded downwards into the trachea. The needle is removed, leaving the guidewire in place. A small skin incision is made and the plastic dilator sheath catheter is advanced over the guidewire. The dilator and guidewire are removed and the sheath left in place. Successive dilators are then used to progressively dilate the tracheal entry point. This enables a relatively large-bore tracheostomy tube to be placed for ventilation. The tube can be changed using a solid stent through the tube to maintain the airway. Good coordination with the anesthetist is important to withdraw the endotracheal tube before entry into the trachea. Care needs to be taken to avoid damage to the endotracheal tube or deflation of the cuff. Hemostasis is usually not a problem. Increased safety of percutaneous mini-tracheostomy insertion using fibreoptic endoscopy involves drawing back the endotracheal tube until it is at cricoid level, and then puncture the anterior trachea at the second tracheal ring interspace under vision. This reduces the risk of puncturing the posterior tracheal wall and paratracheal space or esophagus.

Anatomical Points

The anatomy of the neck is relatively constant in nature, but significant variations can occur with the shape and length of the neck (for example, short thicker "bull necked" individuals), which may impede access and to some degree alter the risk of complications. Large vessels may cross the neck, especially anterior neck veins, and should be identified and ligated. Thyroid enlargement especially of the isthmus, although relatively rare, may also impede access to the trachea. Nerves are usually well away from the site of surgery in the midline and therefore of little risk. Trauma or other surgery to the neck may also alter anatomy and difficulty of access (Table 7.1).

Perspective

The major risk and debility potentially resulting from percutaneous needle mini-tracheostomy surgery is bleeding. This may occasionally lead to a hematoma formation, rarely large enough to require surgical evacuation and hemostasis. Skin necrosis is often very minor and heals spontaneously or with limited dressings. Skin grafts or flaps are rarely required. Infection can rarely be significant. Respiratory obstruction is a potential problem (1) at entry to the trachea as the tracheostomy tube is inserted as the endotracheal tube is withdrawn, (2) later if the endotracheal tube dislodges, (3) at the time of tube changes, or (4) from blood clot or mucus plug obstruction. Excessive cuff pressure may lead to ulceration and tracheal necrosis. Tracheomalacia causes decreased rigidity of the cartilage in the trachea and tracheal collapse. Tracheal stenosis may result from fibrosis/scarring of the tracheal wall. Cosmetic deformity at the tracheostomy site in the central lower neck is common. Accidental puncture of other neck structures: vessels and esophagus, and thyroid tissue can occur, as can tube dislodgement and surgical emphysema.

Table 7.1 Percutaneous mini-tracheostomy estimated frequency of complications, risks, and consequences

Complications, risks, and consequences	Estimated frequency
Most significant/serious complications	
Infection	1–5 %
Bleeding/hematoma formation	1–5 %
Vascular injury	1–5 %
External jugular vein branches	
Thyroid injury[a]	1–5 %
Damage to endotracheal tube/cuff	1–5 %
Respiratory obstruction	
Early or late	1–5 %
Rare significant/serious problems	
Tracheal necrosis[a]	0.1–1 %
Tracheal stenosis[a]	0.1–1 %
Tracheomalacia[a]	0.1–1 %
Neural injury	0.1–1 %
Recurrent laryngeal nerve (X)	
Cervical plexus[a]	
Surgical emphysema (major)	0.1–1 %
Tracheal rupture	<0.1 %
Persistent or recurrent cyst/sinus/fistula	<0.1 %
Less serious complications	
Pain or tenderness (sore throat; sore neck—transient)	
Acute (<4 weeks)	>80 %
Chronic (>12 weeks)	1–5 %
Numbness/altered sensation	1–5 %
Bruising	50–80 %
Dimpling/deformity of the skin	1–5 %
Flap (skin) necrosis (significant)	0.1–1 %
Wound scarring (poor cosmetic result)[a]	1–5 %

[a]Dependent on underlying pathology, anatomy, surgical technique, extent of surgery, and preferences

Major Complications

The most serious complications can arise from **tracheal tube dislodgement** causing **respiratory obstruction**, or **damage to the trachea**. **Oxygen desaturation** at the time of tracheostomy tube insertion can be a major issue if the airway is not maintained. Pre-oxgenation prior to tube insertion/manipulation is helpful in providing more safety and time. **Bleeding** may be significant and reduce vision and difficulty with placement of the tube into the trachea. **Infection** is rarely severe, but **chronic purulent discharge** around the tracheostomy tube entry site is not uncommon. **Abscess formation** and **systemic sepsis** are very rare. **Surgical emphysema** is rarely severe and due to air-leak around the tube into the tissues. **Tracheal ulceration and necrosis** may arise form excessive cuff pressure and prolonged tracheostomy or prior endotracheal intubation. **Tracheal rupture** is very rare. **Tracheal stenosis** may arise from fibrosis and scarring resulting from tracheal ulceration or necrosis.

Cosmetic deformity from the indrawn scar is not uncommon and can be surgically corrected later, but needs to be balanced against the necessity for a tracheostomy.

Consent and Risk Reduction

Main Points to Explain

- GA risk
- Respiratory obstruction
- Bleeding/hematoma
- Wound infection
- Abscess formation
- Cosmetic deformity
- Further surgery

Open Tracheostomy

Description

General anesthesia is almost always used. Local anesthesia may be used on selected occasions with heavy sedation or in the unconscious patient. A transverse or curved skin crease incision in the lower neck is usually used. The fascia between the strap muscles is divided in the midline to expose the thyroid isthmus. The thyroid isthmus is exposed at the second tracheal ring. Curved artery clips are passed beneath the isthmus using gentle dissection to avoid bleeding and the isthmus is clamped either side of the midline to expose the trachea. A square section of the anterior trachea is removed or a flap is created and brought outwards, hinged inferiorly. Good coordination with the anesthetist is important to withdraw the endotracheal tube before entry into the trachea. Care needs to be taken to avoid damage to the endotracheal tube or deflation of the cuff. Hemostasis is ensured using diathermy or occasionally ligatures if needed. Care should be taken to avoid ignition of gases or alcohol from diathermy, where used. A cuffed tracheal tube is inserted.

Anatomical Points

The anatomy of the neck is relatively constant in nature, but significant variations can occur with the shape and length of the neck (for example, short thicker "bull necked" individuals), which may impede access and to some degree alter the risk of complications. Large vessels may cross the neck, especially anterior neck veins and should be identified and ligated. Thyroid enlargement especially of the isthmus, although relatively rare, may also impede access to the trachea. Nerves are usually well away from the site of surgery in the midline and therefore of little risk (Table 7.2).

Table 7.2 Open tracheostomy estimated frequency of complications, risks, and consequences

Complications, risks, and consequences	Estimated frequency
Most significant/serious complications	
Infection	1–5 %
Bleeding/hematoma formation	1–5 %
Vascular injury	1–5 %
External jugular vein branches	
Neural injury	1–5 %
Recurrent laryngeal nerve (X)	
Cervical plexus[a]	
Thyroid injury[a]	1–5 %
Damage to endotracheal tube/cuff	1–5 %
Respiratory obstruction	
Early or late	1–5 %
Rare significant/serious problems	
Tracheal necrosis	0.1–1 %
Tracheal stenosis	0.1–1 %
Tracheomalacia	0.1–1 %
Tracheal rupture	<0.1 %
Surgical emphysema (major)	0.1–1 %
Persistent or recurrent cyst/sinus/fistula	<0.1 %
Less serious complications	
Pain or tenderness (sore throat; sore neck—transient)	
Acute (<4 weeks)	>80 %
Chronic (>12 weeks)	1–5 %
Seroma formation (persistent)	1–5 %
Numbness/altered sensation	1–5 %
Bruising	50–80 %
Dimpling/deformity of the skin	1–5 %
Dehiscence	<0.1 %
Flap (skin) necrosis (significant)	0.1–1 %
Wound scarring (poor cosmetic result)[a]	1–5 %
Drain tube(s)	5–20 %

[a]Dependent on underlying pathology, anatomy, surgical technique, extent of surgery, and preferences

Perspective

The major risk and debility resulting from open tracheostomy surgery is bleeding. This may occasionally lead to a hematoma formation, rarely large enough to require surgical evacuation and hemostasis. Numbness of the neck is uncommon, but can be annoying, making shaving difficult causing injury, or making application of cosmetics difficult. Dehiscence and flap necrosis are often very minor and heal spontaneously or with limited dressings. Skin grafts or flaps are rarely required. Infection can rarely be significant. Respiratory obstruction is a potential problem (1) at entry to the trachea as the tracheostomy tube is inserted as the endotracheal tube is withdrawn, (2) later if the endotracheal tube dislodges and/or the tracheal flap (if used) obstructs the trachea, (3) at the time of tube changes, or (4) from blood clot or mucus plug obstruction. Excessive cuff pressure may lead to ulceration and tracheal necrosis. Tracheomalacia may lead to decreased rigidity of the cartilage in the trachea and tracheal collapse. Tracheal stenosis may result from fibrosis/scarring of the tracheal wall. Cosmetic deformity at the tracheostomy site in the central lower neck is common.

Major Complications

The most serious complications can arise from **tracheal tube dislodgement** causing **respiratory obstruction**, or **damage to the trachea**. **Oxygen desaturation** at the time of tracheostomy tube insertion can be a major issue if the airway is not maintained. Pre-oxgenation prior to tube insertion/manipulation is helpful in providing more safety and time. **Bleeding** may be significant and reduce vision and difficulty with placement of the tube into the trachea. **Infection** is rarely severe, but **chronic purulent discharge** around the tracheostomy tube entry site is not uncommon. **Abscess formation** and **systemic sepsis** are very rare. **Surgical emphysema** is rarely severe and due to air-leak around the tube into the tissues. **Tracheal ulceration and necrosis** may arise from excessive cuff pressure and prolonged tracheostomy or prior endotracheal intubation. **Tracheal rupture** is very rare. **Tracheal stenosis** may arise from fibrosis and scarring resulting from tracheal ulceration or necrosis. **Cosmetic deformity** from the indrawn scar is not uncommon, but needs to be balanced against the necessity for a tracheostomy.

Consent and Risk Reduction

Main Points to Explain

- GA risk
- Respiratory obstruction
- Bleeding/hematoma
- Wound infection
- Abscess formation
- Cosmetic deformity
- Further surgery

Salivary Gland Surgery: Parotid Gland Surgery—Superficial Parotidectomy

Description

General anesthesia is almost always used, and no muscle relaxant, or a shorter acting one is preferred, to permit nerve stimulation. Superficial parotidectomy is removal of the superficial part (lobe) of the parotid gland. An incision is usually made just anteriorly to the ear extending into the upper neck. A pre-tragal lesion within the posterior portion of the gland may utilize a pre-tragal incision alone, allowing facial nerve dissection and tumor excision through a small incision. Lesions which are between the tragus and the angle of the jaw may be removed using a modified "S" incision around the lower ear and onto the neck, again with facial nerve dissection and tumor excision through a relatively small incision. The fine marginal mandibular branch of the facial nerve is usually avoided by keeping the incision at least 2 cm below the mandibular margin. The thin skin overlying the parotid gland is dissected and the flap is raised free from the gland. This procedure aims to dissect the parotid gland with preservation of the facial (VII cranial) nerve. The parotid *duct* branches are intentionally transected during the procedure, branches to the deeper parts of the gland usually remain. Dissection of the skin flap should be between the submuscular aponeurosis and the dermal layer to avoid risk of skin puncture and tumor capsule entry and allows good healing of the flap with excellent cosmetic outcomes. Nerve integrity monitoring can help in training surgeons in parotidectomy and to protect the nerve during dissection to avoid traction, which causes neuropraxia. A nerve stimulator can also confirm preservation of the nerve branches and likely recovery of any neuropraxia. Identification of the main VII nerve trunk arising from the base of the bony auditory canal at the angle with the mastoid, or tracing it back from a branch (an easy anatomical site to find a branch is over the retromandibular vein). Although all accidental injury should ideally be avoided, injury to the branch to orbicularis oculi branch is generally more debilitating than lower branch injuries. The gland is very vascular and oozing of blood is common, together with some salivary fluid leakage. For this reason, a wound drain is often used at completion (Figs. 7.1 and 7.2).

Anatomical Points

Variations in the course facial (VII) nerve are common with variable branching being typical between patients. Careful dissection following the facial nerve branches is usually performed either commencing from the main VII nerve trunk or with the fine branches backwards. A nerve stimulator is sometimes helpful in locating the facial nerve branches, as is the avoidance of long-acting paralyzing agents during anesthesia. Most of the variants of the mandibular branch of the VIIn. course lie within 2 cm of the inferior border of mandible, so that placement of incisions below this level reduces risk of injury. Injury to this branch causes drooping of the mouth on the same side. The zygomatic branch is usually small and can be tortuous. This branch supplies the orbicularis occuli m. and injury causes difficulty with eye closure. The VIIn. main trunk is usually relatively constant in position and found just deep to the bony prominence at the joint with the cartilaginous portion of the external auditory tube. Some neuropraxia of the VIIn. is usual due to the trauma of dissection (Table 7.3).

Fig. 7.1 Malignant parotid mass (melanoma) and facial (VII) nerve palsy

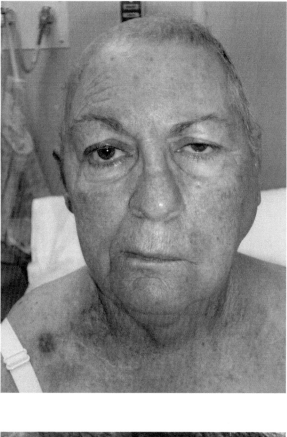

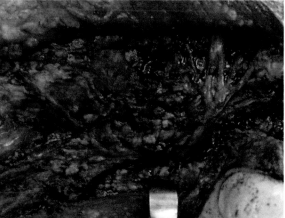

Fig. 7.2 Facial nerve (VII) exposed during a superficial parotidectomy

Table 7.3 Superficial parotidectomy estimated frequency of complications, risks, and consequences

Complications, risks, and consequences		Estimated frequency
Most significant/serious complications		
Infection		1–5 %
Bleeding/hematoma formation		1–5 %
Salivary collection/seroma formation (persistent)		5–20 %
Facial nerve injury	– Overall (all)	20–50 %
	– Permanent major	0.1–1 %
	– Permanent minor	1–5 %
	– Transient	20–50 %
Auriculotemporal syndrome of Frey		
Frey's syndrome (auriculotemporal nerve, facial nerve crossover causing gustatory sweating)		20–50 %
Great auricular nerve injury (Earlobe numbness)[a]		50–80 %
Tumor recurrence (benign or malignant)[b]		1–5 %
Recurrent parotitis[b]		1–5 %
Cyst recurrence[b]		1–5 %
First bite syndrome		5–20 %
Rare significant/serious problems		
Salivary fistula		0.1–1 %
Flap (skin) necrosis (significant)		0.1–1 %
Sympathetic nerve/chain injury (rare) (Horner's syndrome)		<0.1 %
Less serious complications		
Pain or tenderness (sore throat; sore neck—transient)		
Acute (<4 weeks)		20–50 %
Chronic (>12 weeks)		0.1–1 %
Bruising		50–80 %
Numbness/altered sensation		50–80 %
Twitching (facial muscles)		5–20 %
Requirement for skin flaps or grafts[b]		<0.1 %
Dehiscence		<0.1 %
Wound scarring (poor cosmetic result)[b]		1–5 %
Dimpling/deformity of the skin		1–5 %
Drain tube(s)[b]		1–5 %

>80 %; 50–80 %; 20–50 %; 5–20 %; 1–5 %; 0.1–1 %; <0.1 %
[a]Depending on incision type and placement
[b]Dependent on underlying pathology, anatomy, surgical technique, and preferences

Perspective

The major debility resulting from superficial parotidectomy is severe, permanent facial nerve injury resulting in ipsilateral complete facial paralysis. Minor injury to the facial nerve is not uncommon resulting in partial paralysis and facial drooping. Often, this affects one or two branches of the facial nerve and only the muscles supplied by these neural branches are then paralyzed. Minor paralysis or weakness is common and this usually will recover several weeks postoperatively. Residual weakness can be accompanied by twitching of some groups of the facial muscles; however, twitching can continue after recovery of sensory and motor function. Bleeding is usually minor, occasionally leading to a hematoma and rarely large enough to require surgical evacuation and hemostasis. The true frequency of nerve injuries, Frey's syndrome, earlobe numbness, and twitching is difficult to accurately ascertain, since many patients will report a very mild form of these features. When closely examined and questioned, patients will often report short-lived symptoms especially when tired, stressed, or exposed to cold. Frey's syndrome is rare prior to 6 weeks postoperatively and often stops spontaneously by 3–6 months, but topical antiperspirants or subdermal Botox may reduce symptoms of gustatory sweating. Numbness of the earlobe and of the face or neck is common and can be annoying, making shaving difficult causing injury, or making application of cosmetics difficult. First bite syndrome is pain on the initial bite each time when eating, which reduces with each subsequent bite. The true frequency of seromas, salivary collections, and even fistulae is uncertain since many are not reported or transitory (day to weeks) and are not considered significant. If prolonged, these may respond to botox injected into the residual gland. This poses almost no risk to facial nerve function. Dehiscence and flap necrosis are often very minor and heal spontaneously or with limited dressings. Skin grafts or flaps are rarely required. Longer-term complications of parotid gland surgery evolve over time. Recurrence of tumor or inflammation depends on the individual problem and situation. Tumor recurrence is maximal in the first 2 years after surgery, but can occur years after surgery. Wound infections usually occur as an early complication, within the first 3 days.

Major Complications

One of the most serious potential complications are **total or partial facial nerve damage** where all or some branches of the nerve may be affected, which in its most serious form leads to complete paralysis of the facial muscles causing lateral lip drooping, producing drooling, and difficulty closing the eye on the affected side causing occular trauma, keratitis, and corneal ulceration. This can be permanent, but usually partially or completely recovers, depending on the extent of injury. Further surgery may be required to promote eye and mouth closure. **Frey's syndrome** (gustatory sweating) can occasionally be very severe producing excessive sweating with the smell or taste of food and very rarely requires surgical division of the auriculotemporal nerve. When **tumor recurrence** occurs after superficial parotidectomy for a pleomorphic adenoma or malignant tumor, it is typically in the form of multiple cutaneous/subcutaneous nodules. These can usually be excised with or without adjuvant radiotherapy. Radiotherapy or chemotherapy may be recommended for some malignant tumors treated by superficial parotidectomy. **Seroma (or salivary collection) formation** is not uncommon, but usually presents few problems for the patient in the long-term. **Salivary fistula** is rare and often closes spontaneously, but can be a significant problem if it fails to do so and becomes persistent. **Recurrent**

parotitis can be a severe problem following superficial parotidectomy for intractable parotid inflammation. **Severe skin flap necrosis** is very rare because of the excellent vascular supply to the face, but necrosis may rarely require flap repair or free skin grafting. **Horner's syndrome**, although very rare, can cause embarrassment for the patient due to the constricted pupil on the affected side. **Numbness** over the face and/or neck may be unpleasant and make shaving or cosmetic application problematic.

Consent and Risk Reduction

Main Points to Explain

- GA risk
- Respiratory obstruction
- Bleeding/hematoma
- Wound infection
- Abscess formation
- Cosmetic deformity
- Further surgery

Salivary Gland Surgery: Parotid Gland Surgery—Total Parotidectomy

Description

General anesthesia is almost always used, and no muscle relaxant, or a shorter acting one is preferred, to permit nerve stimulation. Total parotidectomy is removal of the entire parotid gland including the superficial and the deep parts (lobes). Total parotidectomy is infrequently performed, usually for tumor resection. A modified "S" incision made just anteriorly and around the lower ear and onto the neck may be used. The facial (VII cranial) nerve may need to be sacrificed if involved with tumor and unable to be retained. The fine marginal mandibular branch of the facial nerve is usually avoided by keeping the incision at least 2 cm below the mandibular margin. The thin skin overlying the parotid gland is dissected and the flap is raised free from the gland. Dissection of the skin flap should be between the submuscular aponeurosis and the dermal layer to avoid risk of skin puncture and tumor capsule entry and allows good healing of the flap with excellent cosmetic outcomes. Nerve integrity monitoring can help in training surgeons in parotidectomy and to protect the nerve during dissection to avoid traction, which causes neuropraxia. A nerve stimulator can also confirm preservation of the nerve branches and likely recovery of any neuropraxia. Identification of the main VII nerve trunk arising from the base of the bony auditory canal at the angle with the mastoid, or tracing it back from a branch (an easy anatomical site to find a branch is over the retromandibular vein). Although all accidental injury should be ideally avoided, injury to the branch to orbicularis oculi branch is generally more debilitating than lower branch injuries. The parotid duct is transected and usually ligated during the procedure. The gland is very vascular and oozing of blood is common. A wound drain is often used at completion. Malignant involvement of the nerve will necessitate sacrifice of involved branches or the entire nerve.

Anatomical Points

Total unilateral facial muscle paralysis occurs if the facial nerve is divided and resected. The smaller, deep part of the parotid gland extends posterior to the ramus of mandible effectively between the external and internal carotid arteries. Variations in the course facial nerve are common with variable branching being typical between patients. If retained, careful dissection following the facial nerve branches is usually performed either commencing from the main VII nerve trunk or sometimes with the fine branches backwards. A nerve stimulator is sometimes helpful in locating the facial nerve branches, as is the avoidance of long-acting paralyzing agents during anesthesia. Most of the variants of the mandibular branch of the VIIn. course lie within 2 cm of the inferior border of mandible, so that placement of incisions below this level reduces risk of injury. Injury to this branch causes drooping of the mouth on the same side. The zygomatic branch is usually small and can be tortuous. This branch supplies the orbicularis occuli m. and injury causes difficulty with eye closure. The VIIn. main trunk is usually relatively constant in position and found just deep to the bony prominence at the joint with the cartilaginous portion of the external auditory tube. Some neuropraxia of the VIIn. is usual due to the trauma of dissection (Table 7.4).

Perspective

The **major** debility potentially resulting from total parotidectomy is severe, permanent **facial nerve injury** resulting in complete ipsilateral facial paralysis. If the nerve is infiltrated with tumor, then the nerve may require to be sacrificed. **Minor** injury to the facial nerve is not uncommon if the nerve is preserved, often arising from extensive dissection, resulting in partial paralysis and facial drooping. This may affect one or more branches of the facial nerve and only the muscles supplied by these neural branches are then paralyzed. Minor paralysis or weakness may recover several weeks postoperatively. Residual weakness can be accompanied by twitching of some groups of the facial muscles; however, **twitching** can continue

Table 7.4 Total parotidectomy estimated frequency of complications, risks, and consequences

Complications, risks, and consequences		Estimated frequency
Most significant/serious complications		
Infection		1–5 %
Bleeding/hematoma formation		1–5 %
Salivary collection/seroma formation (persistent)		5–20 %
Facial nerve injury	– Overall (all)[a]—if preserved	20–50 %
	– Permanent major[a]	1–5 %
	– Permanent minor	5–20 %
	– Transient	20–50 %
	– Complete paralysis—if sacrificed[a]	100 %
Auriculotemporal syndrome of Frey		
Frey's syndrome (auriculotemporal nerve, facial nerve crossover causing gustatory sweating)		20–50 %
Great auricular nerve injury (Earlobe numbness)[a]		50–80 %
Cervical plexus injury[a]		5–20 %
Tumor recurrence (benign or malignant)[a]		1–5 %
Recurrent parotitis[a]		1–5 %
First bite syndrome		5–20 %
Rare significant/serious problems		
Salivary fistula		0.1–1 %
Flap (skin) necrosis (significant)		0.1–1 %
Sympathetic nerve/chain injury (rare) (Horner's syndrome)		<0.1 %
Less serious complications		
Pain or tenderness (sore throat; sore neck—transient)		
Acute (<4 weeks)		20–50 %
Chronic (>12 weeks)		0.1–1 %
Bruising		50–80 %
Numbness/altered sensation		50–80 %
Twitching (facial muscles)		5–20 %
Requirement for skin flaps or grafts[a]		<0.1 %
Dehiscence		<0.1 %
Wound scarring (poor cosmetic result)[a]		1–5 %
Dimpling/deformity of the skin		1–5 %
Drain tube(s)[a]		1–5 %

[a]Dependent on underlying pathology, anatomy, surgical technique, and preferences

after recovery of sensory and motor function. Because dissection for total parotidectomy is often greater than for superficial parotidectomy the relative risk of facial nerve injury is higher. **Bleeding** is usually minor, occasionally leading to a hematoma and rarely large enough to require surgical evacuation and hemostasis. The true frequency of nerve injuries, Frey's syndrome, earlobe numbness, and twitching is difficult to accurately ascertain, since patients will report a very mild form of these features. When closely examined and questioned, patients will often report short-lived symptoms especially when tired, stressed, or exposed to cold. Frey's syndrome is rare prior to 6 weeks postoperatively and often stops spontaneously by 3–6 months, but topical antiperspirants or subdermal Botox may reduce symptoms of gustatory sweating. First bite syndrome is pain on the initial bite each time when eating and reducing with subsequent bites. **Numbness** of the earlobe and of the face or neck is common and can be annoying, making shaving difficult causing injury, or making application of cosmetics difficult. First bite syndrome is pain on the initial bite each time when eating and reducing with subsequent bites. The true frequency of **seromas**, salivary collections, and even fistulae is uncertain since many are not reported or transitory (day to weeks) and are not considered significant. If prolonged, these may respond to botox injected into the residual gland. This poses almost no risk to facial nerve function. Dehiscence and **flap necrosis** are often very minor and heal spontaneously or with limited dressings. Skin grafts or flaps are rarely required. Longer-term complications of parotid gland surgery evolve over time. Recurrence of tumor or inflammation depends on the individual problem and situation. Tumor recurrence is maximal in the first 2 years after surgery, but can occur years after surgery. Wound infections usually occur as an early complication, within the first 3 days.

Major Complications

One of the most serious potential complications is **total or partial facial nerve damage** where all or some branches of the nerve may be affected, which in its most serious form leads to complete paralysis of the facial muscles causing lateral lip drooping, producing drooling, and difficulty closing the eye on the affected side causing occular trauma, keratitis, and corneal ulceration. This can be permanent, but usually partially or completely recovers, depending on the extent of injury. Further surgery may be required to promote eye and mouth closure. **Frey's syndrome** (gustatory sweating) can occasionally be very severe producing excessive sweating with the smell or taste of food and may require surgical division of the auriculotemporal nerve. When **tumor recurrence** occurs after total parotidectomy for a pleomorphic adenoma or malignant tumor, it is typically in the form of multiple cutaneous/subcutaneous nodules, but can be deep towards the skull base. These are usually excised with or without adjuvant radiotherapy. Radiotherapy or chemotherapy may be recommended for some malignant tumors treated by total parotidectomy. **Bleeding** from deep dissection can potentially be major from the carotid arteries or branches. **Seroma (or salivary collection) formation** is not uncommon, but usually presents few problems for the patient in the long-term, **salivary fistula** is rare and often closes spontaneously, but can be a significant problem if it fails to do so and becomes persistent. **Recurrent parotitis** can occur in the residual, accessory or opposite parotid following total unilateral parotidectomy for intractable parotid inflammation. **Severe skin flap necrosis** is very rare because of the excellent vascular supply to the face, but necrosis may rarely require flap repair or free skin grafting. **Horner's syndrome**, although very rare, can cause embarrassment for the patient due to the constricted pupil on the affected side. **Numbness** over the face and/or neck may be unpleasant and make shaving or cosmetic application problematic.

Consent and Risk Reduction

Main Points to Explain

- GA risk
- Respiratory obstruction
- Bleeding/hematoma
- Wound infection
- Abscess formation
- Cosmetic deformity
- Further surgery

Salivary Gland Surgery: Parotid Gland Surgery—Parotid Cyst Excision

Description

General anesthesia is almost always used, and no muscle relaxant, or a shorter act-ing one is preferred, to permit nerve stimulation. Parotid cysts are relatively rare, but simply due to the larger size of the superficial lobe compared to the deep lobe, occur more often in the superficial lobe. The cyst can usually be removed with a narrow cuff of normal surrounding parotid. Paradoxically, although the operation may be smaller than for a superficial lobecomy, a similar sized incision is usually required for access, just anteriorly to the ear extending into the upper neck. Not infrequently, a superficial parotidectomy may be the best operation to perform for cyst removal, especially if large. The facial (VII cranial) nerve may need to be for-mally defined or sometimes can be dissected without displaying the entire proximal nerve. The fine marginal mandibular branch of the facial nerve is usually avoided by keeping the incision at least 2 cm below the mandibular margin. The thin skin over-lying the parotid gland is dissected and the flap is raised free from the gland. This procedure aims to dissect the entire parotid gland. The parotid duct may be encoun-tered and ligated during the procedure. The gland is very vascular and oozing of blood is common. A wound drain is often used at completion.

Anatomical Points

Variations in the course facial nerve are common, with variable branching being typical between patients. Careful dissection following the facial nerve branches is usually performed either commencing from the main VII nerve trunk or sometimes with the fine branches backwards. A nerve stimulator is sometimes helpful in locating the facial nerve branches, as is the avoidance of long-acting paralyzing agents during anesthesia. Most of the variants of the mandibular branch of the VIIn. course lie within 2 cm of the inferior border of mandible, so that placement of incisions below this level reduces risk of injury. Injury to this branch causes drooping of the mouth on the same side. The zygomatic branch is usually small and can be tortuous. This branch supplies the orbicularis occuli m. and injury causes difficulty with eye closure. The VIIn. main trunk is usually relatively constant in position and found just deep to the bony prominence at the joint with the cartilaginous portion of the external auditory tube. Some neuropraxia of the VIIn. is usual due to the trauma of dissection (Table 7.5).

Table 7.5 Parotid cyst excision estimated frequency of complications, risks, and consequences

Complications, risks, and consequences		Estimated frequency
Most significant/serious complications		
Infection		1–5 %
Bleeding/hematoma formation		1–5 %
Salivary collection/seroma formation (persistent)		5–20 %
Cyst recurrence (benign or malignant)[a]		1–5 %
Facial nerve injury	– Overall (all)	20–50 %
	– Permanent major	0.1–1 %
	– Permanent minor	1–5 %
	– Transient	5–20 %
Great auricular nerve injury[a] (Earlobe numbness)		50–80 %
Cervical plexus injury[a]		50–80 %
Auriculotemporal syndrome of Frey[a]		
Frey's syndrome (auriculotemporal nerve, facial nerve crossover causing gustatory sweating)		20–50 %
Rare significant/serious problems		
Salivary fistula		0.1–1 %
Recurrent parotitis[a]		0.1–1 %
Flap (skin) necrosis (significant)		0.1–1 %
Requirement for skin flaps or grafts[a]		<0.1 %
Sympathetic nerve/chain injury (rare) (Horner's syndrome)		<0.1 %
Less serious complications		
Pain or tenderness (sore throat; sore neck—transient)		
Acute (<4 weeks)		20–50 %
Chronic (>12 weeks)		0.1–1 %
Bruising		50–80 %
Numbness/altered sensation		50–80 %
Twitching (facial muscles)		5–20 %
Dehiscence		<0.1 %
Wound scarring (poor cosmetic result)[a]		1–5 %
Dimpling/deformity of the skin		1–5 %
Drain tube(s)[a]		1–5 %

[a]Dependent on underlying pathology, anatomy, surgical technique, extent of surgery, and preferences

Perspective

The major debility potentially resulting from parotid cyst surgery with or without superficial parotidectomy is severe, permanent facial nerve injury resulting in ipsilateral complete facial paralysis. Minor injury to the facial nerve is not uncommon resulting in partial paralysis and facial drooping. Often this affects one or two branches of the facial nerve and only the muscles supplied by these neural branches are then paralyzed. Minor paralysis or weakness is common and this usually will recover several weeks postoperatively. Residual weakness can be accompanied by twitching of some groups of the facial muscles; however, twitching can continue after recovery of sensory and motor function. Bleeding is usually minor, occasionally leading to a hematoma and rarely large enough to require surgical evacuation and hemostasis. The true frequency of nerve injuries, Frey's syndrome, earlobe numbness and twitching is difficult to accurately ascertain, since many patients will report a very mild form of these features. When closely examined and questioned, patients will often report short-lived symptoms especially when tired, stressed, or exposed to cold. Numbness of the earlobe and of the face or neck is common and can be annoying, making shaving difficult causing injury, or making application of cosmetics difficult. The true frequency of seromas, salivary collections, and even fistulae is uncertain, since many are not reported or transitory and are not considered significant. Dehiscence and flap necrosis are often very minor and heal spontaneously or with limited dressings. Skin grafts or flaps are rarely required.

Major Complications

One of the most serious potential complications is **total or partial facial nerve damage** where all or some branches of the nerve may be affected, which in its most serious form leads to complete paralysis of the facial muscles causing lateral lip drooping, producing drooling, and difficulty closing the eye on the affected side causing occular trauma, keratitis, and corneal ulceration. This can be permanent, but usually partially or completely recovers, depending on the extent of injury. Further surgery may be required to promote eye and mouth closure. **Frey's syndrome** (gustatory sweating) can occasionally be very severe producing excessive sweating with the smell or taste of food and may require surgical division of the auriculotemporal nerve. **Cyst recurrence** may occur after partial parotidectomy, either in the deep or any remaining superficial lobe. These are usually able to be excised by repeat surgery, depending on the location. **Seroma (or salivary collection) formation** is not uncommon, but usually presents few problems for the patient in the long-term, **salivary fistula** is rare and often closes spontaneously, but can be a significant problem if it fails to do so and becomes persistent. **Recurrent parotitis** is rare, but can be a severe problem in some cases. **Severe skin flap necrosis** is very rare because of the excellent vascular supply to the face, but necrosis may rarely require flap repair or free skin grafting. **Horner's syndrome**, although very rare, can cause embarrass-ment for the patient due to the constricted pupil on the affected side.

Consent and Risk Reduction

Main Points to Explain

- GA risk
- Respiratory obstruction
- Bleeding/hematoma
- Wound infection
- Abscess formation
- Cosmetic deformity
- Further surgery

Salivary Gland Surgery: Submandibular Gland Surgery—Submandibular Gland Excision

Description

General anesthesia is almost always used. The transverse "skin crease" incision in the upper neck is usually used. The fine marginal mandibular branch of the facial nerve is usually avoided by keeping the incision at least 2 cm below the mandibular margin. A flap of skin and subcutaneous tissue is raised just deep to the platysma muscle, to locate the submandibular gland just deep to the mandible. This procedure aims to dissect the entire submandibular gland. The submandibular duct is encountered and ligated during the procedure, avoiding associated nerves. The gland is very vascular and some minor oozing of blood is common. Asking the anesthetist to perform a valsalva will expose any small veins that are in spasm, or covered by clot and to allow ligation of these prior to wound closure. A wound drain is often used at completion.

Anatomical Points

The submandibular gland lies against the deep inferior aspect of lateral arch of mandible, with the submandibular duct exiting forwards to open into the floor of the anterior mouth, just posterior to the front lower incisors and lateral to the frenulum. The lingual nerve [lingual branch of the trigeminal (V) cranial nerve] winds around the submandibular duct deep to the gland, and the hypoglossal (XII) cranial nerve lies deep to the digastric muscle central tendon, again deep to and below the submandibular gland. Variations in the course facial (VII) cranial nerve are common, with variable branching being typical between patients. Most of the variants of the mandibular branch of the VIIn. course lie within 2 cm of the inferior border of mandible, so that placement of incisions below this level reduces risk of injury. An incision placed along the anterior edge of the sternomastoid, or laterally in the line of the hyoid, is usually safer and cosmetic. Dividing the platysma close to the sternomastoid and elevating the submandibular fascia dissects below the marginal mandibular nerve. Injury to this branch causes drooping of the mouth on the same side. Some minor neuropraxia of the VIIn. is not uncommon, resulting from retraction and the trauma of dissection. Maintaining the cervical branch of VII preserves the inferior pull of platysma, stabilizing the lower lip in the act of smiling. This is a different deformity to the depressor muscle dysfunction. The facial artery and vein insinuate and groove the gland giving off small branches, which can be ligated or diathermied. Occasionally the main vessels require ligation, especially in inflammation or malignancy. Inferior gland retraction brings the lingual nerve into view for preservation. Where the submandibular duct and nerve cross, retained stones are not uncommon, with associated inflammation. Of note the hypoglossal nerve often lies immediately deep to the duct at this point, posing risk of injury. Bleeding vessels should be separated from the nerve before attempting hemostasis (Table 7.6).

Table 7.6 Submandibular gland excision estimated frequency of complications, risks, and consequences

Complications, risks, and consequences		Estimated frequency
Most significant/serious complications		
Infection		1–5 %
Bleeding/hematoma formation		1–5 %
Vascular injury		
Facial artery and vein[a]		>80 %
Retromandibular vein		5–20 %
Retained duct calculus		1–5 %
Salivary collection/seroma formation (persistent)		5–20 %
Cervical plexus injury[b]		1–5 %
Rare significant/serious problems		
Neural injury	– Mandibular branch of facial nerve[c]	0.1–1 %
	– Lingual nerve (taste)	<0.1 %
	– Hypoglossal nerve (tongue movement)	<0.1 %
Facial nerve injury[c]	– Overall (all)	0.1–1 %
	– Permanent major	<0.1 %
	– Permanent minor	<0.1 %
	– Transient	0.1–1 %

Table 7.6 (continued)

Complications, risks, and consequences	Estimated frequency
Salivary fistula	<0.1 %
Flap (skin) necrosis (significant)	0.1–1 %
Less serious complications	
Pain or tenderness (sore throat; sore neck—transient)	
Acute (<4 weeks)	20–50 %
Chronic (>12 weeks)	0.1–1 %
Bruising	50–80 %
Numbness/altered sensation	1–5 %
Dehiscence	<0.1 %
Dimpling/deformity of the skin	1–5 %
Wound scarring (poor cosmetic result)[b]	1–5 %
Drain tube(s)[b]	1–5 %

[a]The facial vessels are not infrequently ligated in the course of surgery
[b]Dependent on underlying pathology, anatomy, surgical technique, extent of surgery, and preferences
[c]Facial nerve injury is subdivided further for convenience

Perspective

The major debility and risk resulting from submandibular gland surgery is nerve injury, principally to facial, lingual, or hypoglossal nerves. Minor injury to the facial nerve is not common, but can result in partial paralysis and facial drooping, which will usually recover several weeks postoperatively. Residual weakness can be accompanied by twitching of some groups of the facial muscles; however, twitching can continue after recovery of sensory and motor function. Bleeding is usually minor, occasionally leading to a hematoma and rarely large enough to require surgical evacuation and hemostasis. The true frequency of nerve injuries and twitching is difficult to accurately ascertain, since many patients will report only a very mild form of these features. When closely examined and questioned, patients may report short-lived symptoms especially when tired, stressed, or exposed to cold. Numbness of the face or neck is uncommon, but can be annoying, making shaving difficult causing injury, or making application of cosmetics difficult. The true frequency of seromas, salivary collections, and even fistulae is uncertain since many are not reported or transitory and are not considered significant. Dehiscence and flap necrosis are often very minor and heal spontaneously or with limited dressings. Skin grafts or flaps are rarely required (Fig. 7.3).

Major Complications

One of the most serious complications is **damage to the mandibular branch of the facial nerve**, which in its most serious form leads to lateral lip drooping, producing drooling. This can be permanent, but usually partially or completely recovers,

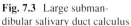

Fig. 7.3 Large submandibular salivary duct calculus

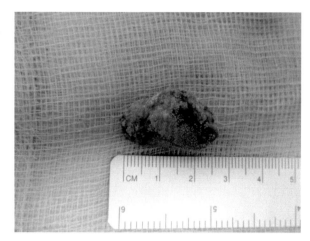

depending on the extent of injury. Further surgery may be required to promote
mouth closure. Injury to the hypoglossal nerve can cause tongue mobility problems,
which can interfere with talking or eating. Lingual nerve injury may result in loss of
taste to the anterior 2/3 of the ipsilateral tongue. **Retained Duct Calculi** rarely
cause problems, but may need surgical removal later. **Seroma (or salivary collection) formation** is not uncommon, but usually presents few problems for the patient
in the long-term, **salivary fistula** is rare and often closes spontaneously, but can be
a significant problem if it fails to do so and becomes persistent. **Skin flap necrosis**
is very rare because of the excellent vascular supply to the neck, but necrosis may
rarely require flap repair or free skin grafting. **Horner's syndrome**, although
exceedingly rare, can cause embarrassment for the patient due to the constricted
pupil on the affected side.

Consent and Risk Reduction

Main Points to Explain

- GA risk
- Respiratory obstruction
- Bleeding/hematoma
- Wound infection
- Abscess formation
- Cosmetic deformity
- Further surgery

Salivary Gland Surgery: Submandibular Gland Surgery—Submandibular Duct Dilatation ± Calculus Removal

Description

Local anesthetic or general anesthetic can be used. The aim is to dilate the opening of the submandibular duct to permit drainage of pus and/or a calculus within the submandibular duct. A removable "stay" suture is usually placed around the duct to prevent the calculus slipping more deeply into the duct, while dilatation is being performed. A dilator, probe, and sometimes a small incision may be used to open the duct orifice. Inflammation and infection may already be established and can increase the risk of "postoperative" infection. Usually, relief of obstruction and anti-biotics settles any infection rapidly.

Anatomical Points

The submandibular duct opens into the anterior floor of the mouth just lateral to the frenulum of the tongue. The normal duct orifice is usually raised slightly as a small papilla, but when inflamed, the opening can be raised and red. Occasionally, the calculus may be palpable and visible within the raised papilla, or more commonly palpable in the floor of mouth. The lingual nerve is generally deep to the floor of mouth as it winds around the submandibular duct; however, it may be injured during deep incision along the duct in order to release a calculus (Table 7.7).

Perspective

Dilatation of the submandibular duct is usually a small very low risk procedure. Infection risk is higher if preexisting infection is present, either subclinically or overtly. Bleeding is not usually serious or common, but some minor oozing is not uncommon, which usually settles spontaneously, unless poor coagulation is present. Occasionally, the calculus can move retrogradely in the duct back towards the sub-mandibular gland, or sometimes can be passed without symptoms just prior to sur-gery. Often the stone can be "milked" distally down the duct towards the opening and then secured with a suture underneath the duct to prevent the calculus refluxing back up the duct during extraction. Extraction often requires incision of the duct opening. Failure to remove the stone is a possibility, and scarring of the opening can occur following dilatation and/or incision or meatotomy. Further later obstruction may occur due to these. Reformation of another calculus can also occur. Long-term pain is well reported as an association with submandibular surgery and problems.

Table 7.7 Submandibular duct dilatation estimated frequency of complications, risks, and consequences

Complications, risks, and consequences	Estimated frequency
Most significant/serious complications[a]	
Infection—overall (mouth, face, gland)	1–5 %
Submandibular duct stenosis	1–5 %
Recurrent submandibular obstruction	1–5 %
Retained duct calculus	1–5 %
Recurrent submandibular calculi	5–20 %
Gustatory (eating) pain	1–5 %
Rare significant/serious problems[a]	
Bleeding/hematoma formation	0.1–1 %
Neural injury – Lingual nerve	<0.1 %
Less serious complications[a]	
Pain or tenderness (sore throat; sore neck—transient)	
Acute (<4 weeks)	5–20 %
Chronic (>12 weeks)	0.1–1 %
Scarring	0.1–1 %
Recurrent surgery	0.1–1 %

[a]Dependent on underlying pathology, anatomy, surgical technique, extent of surgery, and preferences

Major Complications

The **major** risk is cellulitis or systemic infection from an infected, obstructed duct. **Bleeding** is usually minor, except in anticoagulated patients or with a coagulopathy. **Injury to the lingual nerve** injury may result in loss of taste to the anterior 2/3 of the ipsilateral tongue. **Persistent drainage of pus** into the mouth can occur and is unpleasant. **Retained or recurrent calculi** can occur. **Ductal stenosis and recurrent pain** may also occur.

Consent and Risk Reduction

Main Points to Explain

- GA risk
- Bleeding/hematoma
- Wound infection
- Abscess formation
- Recurrent/retained calculi
- Further surgery

Branchial Cyst/Sinus Excision

Description

General anesthesia is almost always used. An oblique or transverse incision in the upper- to mid-neck is usually used as for a selective neck dissection, aiming to protect the marginal mandibular branch of the facial (VII) nerve. Branchial cysts, sinuses, and fistulae are a group of conditions arising from embryological structures that persist beyond birth and often into adulthood. The nature and extent of surgery is largely determined by the type of cyst and/or sinus/fistula that is present, and the type of problem it is causing. The aim is excision of all of the cyst wall and tissue lining the sinus or fistula, usually with primary closure. A wound drain is often used at completion. Malignancy may be a differential diagnosis and this should be considered and kept in mind, where appropriate, to plan for a full neck lymph node dissection, if required. A branchial cyst is effectively a diagnosis of exclusion, as squamous cell carcinoma (SCC) is more common. Mis-diagnosis of a primary oropharyngeal carcinoma with cervical metastasis should be reduced by utilizing CT scans, fine needle biopsy, and panendoscopy prior to neck surgery. Careful planned oncological surgery is important for SCC, whereas more limited localized surgery can be used for branchial cyst/sinus surgery. Using a Valsalva maneuver before closure may identify bleeding points. If pathology examination identifies SCC, a formal oropharyngeal examination, radiologic exam, panendoscopy, and biopsy, with a completion modified radical neck dissection should be performed (Figs. 7.4 and 7.5.)

Anatomical Points

Branchial cysts, sinuses, and fistulae arise from remnants of the second branchial groove and the second branchial cleft (which forms part of the cervical sinus). A cyst may exist alone as a remnant, or may drain via a sinus *internally* into the

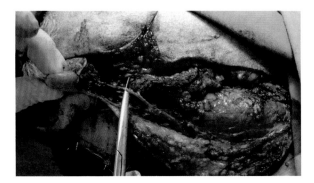

Fig. 7.4 Great auricular nerve preserved during a modified radical neck dissection

Fig. 7.5 Surgical exposure of the accessory (XI) nerve during sentinel node biopsy of the neck

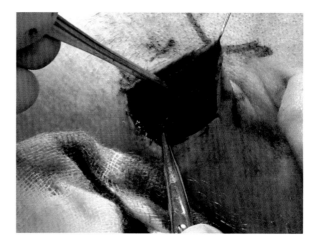

tonsillar fossa (derived from the second pharyngeal pouch), or *externally* via an opening to the anterior neck skin. Rarely, a track (with or without a cyst) may form from the tonsillar fossa epithelium to the skin externally—a *branchial fistula*. Cysts and the fistula may be lined with epithelium also. The path that a fistula usually follows travels between the external and internal carotid arteries, therefore associated anatomically with the internal jugular vein, vagus (X) nerve, recurrent laryngeal nerve, cervical plexus, hypoglossal (XII) nerve, lingual (V) nerve, and sympathetic chain. Deep or complex surgical dissection may also involve the phrenic nerve or upper brachial plexus. Retraction may also place pressure on the mandibular branch of the facial (VII) nerve and submandibular gland. It is critical to identify the greater auricular nerve. Superiorly, the posterior belly of digastric should be identified and followed towards the mastoid. The accessory nerve should be dissected avoiding nerve traction injury. The hypoglossal nerve passes over the external carotid artery and branches, and the branchial sinus tract passes internally between the internal and external carotid arteries between the superior and middle constrictor muscles to the tonsillar fossa. The vagus nerve is identified prior to ligation of the proximal end of the sinus tract. Preservation of the descendens hypoglossi nerve maintains strap muscle function, normal swallowing, and voice function. Inflammatory cyst adherence to the internal jugular vein necessitates venous control on either side to avoid bleeding (Table 7.8).

Perspective

The **major** risk and debility resulting from branchial cyst/sinus/fistula surgery is possible nerve injury, principally to the lingual, facial, recurrent laryngeal, accessory, or hypoglossal nerves. This depends largely on the nature, location, and fixity due to inflammation and scarring. Branchial anomalies are relatively rare entities

Table 7.8 Branchial cyst/sinus excision estimated frequency of complications, risks, and consequences

Complications, risks, and consequences	Estimated frequency
Most significant/serious complications	
Infection	1–5 %
Bleeding/hematoma formation	1–5 %
Vascular injury	1–5 %
Facial artery and vein	
Retromandibular vein	
Internal carotid artery	
External carotid artery	
Internal jugular vein	
External jugular vein	
Neural injury—overall	5–20 %
Mandibular branch of facial (VII) nerve[a]	
Hypoglossal nerve (XII; tongue movement)	
Vagus nerve (X)	
Superior or recurrent laryngeal nerve (X)	
Sympathetic chain[a]	
Cervical plexus[a]	
Accessory (XI) nerve	
Thyroid injury[a]	1–5 %
Rare significant/serious problems	
Voice changes, Horner's syndrome, facial weakness	0.1–1 %
Flap (skin) necrosis (significant)	0.1–1 %
Thoracic duct injury[b]	<0.1 %
Lingual (V) nerve (taste)	<0.1 %
Persistent or recurrent cyst/sinus/fistula	<0.1 %
Less serious complications	
Pain or tenderness (sore throat; sore neck—transient)	
Acute (<4 weeks)	20–50 %
Chronic (>12 weeks)	0.1–1 %
Seroma formation (persistent)	5–20 %
Numbness/altered sensation	1–5 %
Bruising	50–80 %
Dehiscence	<0.1 %
Dimpling/deformity of the skin	1–5 %
Wound scarring (poor cosmetic result)[a]	1–5 %
Drain tube(s)	5–20 %

[a]Dependant on underlying pathology, anatomy, surgical technique, extent of surgery, and preferences
[b]Very rare, but can occur particularly with low left side neck dissections

and this fact itself adds to the relative surgical risk to some degree. **Minor** injury to the facial nerve is also possible, but can result in partial paralysis and facial drooping, which will usually recover several weeks postoperatively. Residual weakness can be accompanied by twitching of some groups of the facial muscles; however, **twitching** can continue after recovery of sensory and motor function. **Bleeding** is usually minor, occasionally leading to a hematoma and rarely large enough to require surgical evacuation and hemostasis. Serious injury to the common, external or internal carotid arteries may also be significant, but rarely leads to major effects such as cerebrovascular injury. The true frequency of nerve injuries and twitching is difficult to accurately ascertain, since patients may report only a very mild form of these features. When closely examined and questioned, patients may report short-lived symptoms especially when tired, stressed, or exposed to cold. **Numbness** of the face or neck is uncommon, but can be annoying, making shaving difficult causing injury, or making application of cosmetics difficult. The true frequency of **seromas**, salivary collections, and even fistulae is uncertain since many are not reported or transitory and are not considered significant. Dehiscence and **flap necrosis** are often very minor and heal spontaneously or with limited dressings. Skin grafts or flaps are rarely required. **Infection** can rarely be significant.

Major Complications

The most serious complications can arise from **damage to one of the cranial nerves [V, VII, X–XII] or phrenic nerve**, or from **internal carotid arterial injury**, which may potentially cause **cerebral infarction** as one of the most severe sequelae. Lingual nerve injury may result in **loss of taste** to the anterior 2/3 of the ipsilateral tongue. **Injury to the mandibular branch of the facial nerve**, in its most serious form, leads to lateral **lip drooping**, producing drooling. If permanent, further surgery may be required to promote mouth closure. Injury to the recurrent laryngeal nerve may cause a **hoarse voice**. **Shoulder droop** may result from accessory nerve injury. **Hypoglossal nerve** injury may cause difficulty with tongue movements for speech and eating. **Seroma (or salivary collection) formation** is not uncommon, but usually presents few problems for the patient in the long-term. **Skin flap necrosis** is very rare because of the excellent vascular supply to the neck, but necrosis may rarely require flap repair or free skin grafting. **Horner's syndrome**, although exceedingly rare, can cause embarrassment for the patient due to the constricted pupil on the affected side. **Recurrence of branchial cyst/sinus/fistula** is reported, presumably due to some residual or separate tissue from the cyst wall and may require further surgery.

Consent and Risk Reduction

Main Points to Explain

- GA risk
- Bleeding/hematoma

- Wound infection
- Abscess formation
- Respiratory obstruction
- Voice changes
- Facial weakness
- Speech/taste changes
- Cosmetic deformity
- Further surgery

Salivary Gland Surgery: Mucous Cyst Excision—Excision of Mucous Cyst of Lip/Cheek

Description

Local anesthetic or general anesthetic may be used. The aim is to excise the cyst wall completely including a small cuff of normal lip mucosa tissue and close the wound directly using either inverted soluble sutures or more rarely a mucosal flap repair.

Anatomical Points

Mucous cysts typically occur in the mucosa of the lower lip as raised, smooth, rounded superficial masses 0.5–2 cm in diameter. They arise from obstructed mucous glands of the lip mucosa, often as a result of local trauma and scarring. The trauma may be due to teeth, dentures, or playing a musical (wind) instrument (Table 7.9).

Table 7.9 Mucous cyst excision of lip/cheek estimated frequency of complications, risks, and consequences

Complications, risks, and consequences	Estimated frequency
Most significant/serious complications[a]	
Recurrence	1–5 %
Rare significant/serious problems[a]	
Infection	0.1–1 %
Bleeding/hematoma formation	0.1–1 %
Neural injury—small labial branches of trigeminal nerve	0.1–1 %
Less serious complications	
Pain or tenderness (sore throat; sore neck—transient)	
Acute (<4 weeks)	5–20 %
Chronic (>12 weeks)	<0.1 %
Wound scarring (poor cosmesis) or dimpling	0.1–1 %

[a]Dependent on underlying pathology, anatomy, surgical technique, and preferences

Perspective

Excision of a mucous cyst is usually a small and very low-risk procedure. Recurrence may occur, as can development of separate cysts in adjacent mucosa, which are difficult to discern from each other. The predisposing or causative factor(s) are often still present.

Major Complications

The major risk is **recurrence** or re-occurrence may necessitate repeated surgery. **Local infection** of the excision site is rare, which very rarely can proceed to cellulitis or even systemic infection, occurring almost exclusively in immunocompromised individuals. **Dehiscence** of the wound may occur, leaving a small ulcer that normally heals within a week. **Bleeding** is usually minor, except perhaps in anticoagulated patients. Rarely, when mucous cysts are removed from the inner cheek mucosa, scarring may obstruct the parotid duct opening causing pain and swelling. Injury to the small sensory nerves is usually not a significant issue, but can cause **numbness**.

Consent and Risk Reduction

Main Points to Explain

- GA risk
- Recurrent cysts
- Bleeding/hematoma
- Wound infection
- Abscess formation
- Further surgery

Further Reading, References, and Resources

Percutaneous Mini-Tracheostomy

Clemente CD. Anatomy – a regional atlas of the human body. 4th ed. Baltimore: Williams and Wilkins; 1997.

Hsiao J, Pacheco-Fowler V. Videos in clinical medicine. Cricothyroidotomy. N Engl J Med. 2008; 358(22):e25.

Jamieson GG. The anatomy of general surgical operations. 2nd ed. Edinburgh: Churchill Livingston; 2006.

Jenvrin J, Pean D. Cricothyroidotomy. N Engl J Med. 2008;359(10):1073.

Pierce RB. "Mini-tracheostomy" with a large-gauge needle. N Engl J Med. 1978;298(18):1036.

Open Tracheostomy

Chan TC, Vilke GM, Bramwell KJ, Davis DP, Hamilton RS, Rosen P. Comparison of wire-guided cricothyrotomy versus standard surgical cricothyrotomy technique. J Emerg Med. 1999; 17:957–62.

Clemente CD. Anatomy –a regional atlas of the human body. 4th ed. Baltimore: Williams and Wilkins; 1997.

Hsiao J, Pacheco-Fowler V. Videos in clinical medicine. Cricothyroidotomy. N Engl J Med. 2008; 358(22):e25.

Jamieson GG. The anatomy of general surgical operations. 2nd ed. Edinburgh: Churchill Livingston; 2006.

Jenvrin J, Pean D. Cricothyroidotomy. N Engl J Med. 2008;359(10):1073.

Pierce RB. "Mini-tracheostomy" with a large-gauge needle. N Engl J Med. 1978;298(18):1036.

Schaumann N, Lorenz V, Schellongowski P, et al. Evaluation of Seldinger technique emergency cricothyroidotomy versus standard surgical cricothyroidotomy in 200 cadavers. Anesthesiology. 2005;102:7–11.

Wong DT, Prabhu AJ, Coloma M, Imasogie N, Chung FF. What is the minimum training required for successful cricothyroidotomy? A study in mannequins. Anesthesiology. 2003;98:349–53.

Superficial Parotidectomy

Al Salamah SM, Khalid K, Khan IA, Gul R. Outcome of surgery for parotid tumours: 5-year experience of a general surgical unit in a teaching hospital. ANZ J Surg. 2005;75(11):948–52.

Bhide SA, Miah A, Barbachano Y, Harrington KJ, Newbold K, Nutting CM. Radical radiotherapy for treatment of malignant parotid tumours: a single centre experience 1995–2005. Br J Oral Maxillofac Surg. 2009;47(4):284–9.

Bova R, Saylor A, Coman WB. Parotidectomy: review of treatment and outcomes. ANZ J Surg. 2004;74(7):563–8.

Chew YK, Noorizan Y, Khir A, Brito-Mutunayagam S. Parotid mass: a 5-year review of parotid surgery. Med J Malaysia. 2007;62(5):388–9.

Chiu AG, Cohen JI, Burningham AR, Andersen PE, Davidson BJ. First bite syndrome: a complication of surgery involving the parapharyngeal space. Head Neck. 2002;24(11):996–9.

Clemente CD. Anatomy –a regional atlas of the human body. 4th ed. Baltimore: Williams and Wilkins; 1997.

Dulguerov P, Quinodoz D, Cosendai G, Piletta P, Marchal F, Lehmann W. Prevention of Frey syndrome during parotidectomy. Arch Otolaryngol Head Neck Surg. 1999;125(8):833–9.

Foghsgaard S, Foghsgaard J, Homøe P. Early post-operative morbidity after superficial parotidectomy: a prospective study concerning pain and resumption of normal activity. Clin Otolaryngol. 2007;32(1):54–7.

Guntinas-Lichius O, Gabriel B, Klussmann JP. Risk of facial palsy and severe Frey's syndrome after conservative parotidectomy for benign disease: analysis of 610 operations. Acta Otolaryngol. 2006;126(10):1104–9.

Iyer NG, Clark JR, Murali R, Gao K, O'Brien CJ. Outcomes following parotidectomy for metastatic squamous cell carcinoma with microscopic residual disease: implications for facial nerve preservation. Head Neck. 2009;31(1):21–7.

Jamieson GG. The anatomy of general surgical operations. 2nd ed. Edinburgh: Churchill Livingston; 2006.

Lin CC, Tsai MH, Huang CC, Hua CH, Tseng HC, Huang ST. Parotid tumors: a 10-year experience. Am J Otolaryngol. 2008;29(2):94–100.

Linkov G, Morris LG, Shah JP, Kraus DH. First bite syndrome: incidence, risk factors, treatment, and outcomes. Laryngoscope. 2012;122(8):1773–8.

Luna-Ortiz K, Sansón-RíoFrío JA, Mosqueda-Taylor A. Frey syndrome. A proposal for evaluating severity. Oral Oncol. 2004;40(5):501–5.

Mavrikakis I. Facial nerve palsy: anatomy, etiology, evaluation, and management. Orbit. 2008;27(6):466–74 (review).

Meier JD, Wenig BL, Manders EC, Nenonene EK. Continuous intraoperative facial nerve monitoring in predicting postoperative injury during parotidectomy. Laryngoscope. 2006; 116(9):1569–72

Mohammed F, Asaria J, Payne RJ, Freeman JL. Retrospective review of 242 consecutive patients treated surgically for parotid gland tumours. J Otolaryngol Head Neck Surg. 2008; 37(3):340–6.

Nouraei SA, Ismail Y, Ferguson MS, McLean NR, Milner RH, Thomson PJ, Welch AR. Analysis of complications following surgical treatment of benign parotid disease. ANZ J Surg. 2008;78(3):134–8.

O'Brien CJ. Current management of benign parotid tumors – the role of limited superficial parotidectomy. Head Neck. 2003;25(11):946–52.

O'Regan B, Bharadwaj G, Elders A. Techniques for dissection of the facial nerve in benign parotid surgery: a cross specialty survey of oral and maxillofacial and ear nose and throat surgeons in the UK. Br J Oral Maxillofac Surg. 2008;46(7):564–6.

Patel RS, Low TH, Gao K, O'Brien CJ. Clinical outcome after surgery for 75 patients with parotid sialadenitis. Laryngoscope. 2007;117(4):644–7.

Picon AI, Coit DG, Shaha AR, Brady MS, Boyle JO, Singh BB, Wong RJ, Busam KJ, Shah JP, Kraus DH. Sentinel lymph node biopsy for cutaneous head and neck melanoma: mapping the parotid gland. Ann Surg Oncol. 2006; (Epub ahead of print).

Redaelli de Zinis LO, Piccioni M, Antonelli AR, Nicolai P. Management and prognostic factors of recurrent pleomorphic adenoma of the parotid gland: personal experience and review of the literature. Eur Arch Otorhinolaryngol. 2008;265(4):447–52.

Roh JL, Kim HS, Park CI. Randomized clinical trial comparing partial parotidectomy versus superficial or total parotidectomy. Br J Surg. 2007;94(9):1081–7.

Ryan WR, Fee WE. Long-term great auricular nerve morbidity after sacrifice during parotidectomy. Laryngoscope. 2009;119(6):1140–6.

Ryan WR, Fee Jr WE. Great auricular nerve morbidity after nerve sacrifice during parotidectomy. Arch Otolaryngol Head Neck Surg. 2006;132(6):642–9.

Santos RC, Chagas JF, Bezerra TF, Baptistella JE, Pagani MA, Melo AR. Frey syndrome prevalence after partial parotidectomy. Braz J Otorhinolaryngol. 2006;72(1):112–5.

Smith JA, Fleming WB. An approach to malignant parotid tumours. Aust N Z J Surg. 1989; 59(4):317–20.

Smith SL, Komisar A. Limited parotidectomy: the role of extracapsular dissection in parotid gland neoplasms. Laryngoscope. 2007;117(7):1163–7.

Suen DT, Chow TL, Lam CY, Wong ES, Lam SH. Sensation recovery improved by great auricular nerve preservation in parotidectomy: a prospective double-blind study. ANZ J Surg. 2007;77(5):374–6.

Umapathy N, Holmes R, Basavaraj S, Roux R, Cable HR. Performance of parotidectomy in non-specialist centers. Arch Otolaryngol Head Neck Surg. 2003;129(9):925–8; discussion 928. (review)

Witt RL. The incidence and management of siaolocele after parotidectomy. Otolaryngol Head Neck Surg. 2009;140(6):871–4.

Zbar AP, Hill AD, Shering SG, Rafferty MA, Moriarty M, McDermott EW, O'Higgins NJ. A 25 year review of parotid surgery. Ir Med J. 1997;90(6):228–30.

Total Parotidectomy

Al Salamah SM, Khalid K, Khan IA, Gul R. Outcome of surgery for parotid tumours: 5-year experience of a general surgical unit in a teaching hospital. ANZ J Surg. 2005;75(11): 948–52.

Bova R, Saylor A, Coman WB. Parotidectomy: review of treatment and outcomes. ANZ J Surg. 2004;74(7):563–8.

Chew YK, Noorizan Y, Khir A, Brito-Mutunayagam S. Parotid mass: a 5-year review of parotid surgery. Med J Malaysia. 2007;62(5):388–9.

Clemente CD. Anatomy –a regional atlas of the human body. 4th ed. Baltimore: Williams and Wilkins; 1997.

Dulguerov P, Quinodoz D, Cosendai G, Piletta P, Marchal F, Lehmann W. Prevention of Frey syndrome during parotidectomy. Arch Otolaryngol Head Neck Surg. 1999;125(8):833–9.

Iyer NG, Clark JR, Murali R, Gao K, O'Brien CJ. Outcomes following parotidectomy for metastatic squamous cell carcinoma with microscopic residual disease: implications for facial nerve preservation. Head Neck. 2009;31(1):21–7.

Jamieson GG. The anatomy of general surgical operations. 2nd ed. Edinburgh: Churchill Livingston; 2006.

Lin CC, Tsai MH, Huang CC, Hua CH, Tseng HC, Huang ST. Parotid tumors: a 10-year experience. Am J Otolaryngol. 2008;29(2):94–100.

Luna-Ortiz K, Sansón-RíoFrío JA, Mosqueda-Taylor A. Frey syndrome. A proposal for evaluating severity. Oral Oncol. 2004;40(5):501–5.

Mavrikakis I. Facial nerve palsy: anatomy, etiology, evaluation, and management. Orbit. 2008; 27(6):466–74 (review)

Meier JD, Wenig BL, Manders EC, Nenonene EK. Continuous intraoperative facial nerve monitoring in predicting postoperative injury during parotidectomy. Laryngoscope. 2006;116(9): 1569–72.

Mohammed F, Asaria J, Payne RJ. Freeman JL. Retrospective review of 242 consecutive patients treated surgically for parotid gland tumours. J Otolaryngol Head Neck Surg. 2008;37(3): 340–6.

Patel RS, Low TH, Gao K, O'Brien CJ. Clinical outcome after surgery for 75 patients with parotid sialadenitis. Laryngoscope. 2007;117(4):644–7.

Picon AI, Coit DG, Shaha AR, Brady MS, Boyle JO, Singh BB, Wong RJ, Busam KJ, Shah JP, Kraus DH. Sentinel lymph node biopsy for cutaneous head and neck melanoma: mapping the parotid gland. Ann Surg Oncol. 2006; (Epub ahead of print).

Roh JL, Kim HS, Park CI. Randomized clinical trial comparing partial parotidectomy versus superficial or total parotidectomy. Br J Surg. 2007;94(9):1081–7.

Ryan WR, Fee Jr WE. Great auricular nerve morbidity after nerve sacrifice during parotidectomy. Arch Otolaryngol Head Neck Surg. 2006;132(6):642–9.

Smith JA, Fleming WB. An approach to malignant parotid tumours. Aust N Z J Surg. 1989;59(4):317–20.

Smith SL, Komisar A. Limited parotidectomy: the role of extracapsular dissection in parotid gland neoplasms. Laryngoscope. 2007;117(7):1163–7.

Suen DT, Chow TL, Lam CY, Wong ES, Lam SH. Sensation recovery improved by great auricular nerve preservation in parotidectomy: a prospective double-blind study. ANZ J Surg. 2007;77(5): 374–6.

Umapathy N, Holmes R, Basavaraj S, Roux R, Cable HR. Performance of parotidectomy in nonspecialist centers. Arch Otolaryngol Head Neck Surg. 2003;129(9):925–8; discussion 928 (review)

Zbar AP, Hill AD, Shering SG, Rafferty MA, Moriarty M, McDermott EW, O'Higgins NJ. A 25 year review of parotid surgery. Ir Med J. 1997;90(6):228–30.

Parotid Cyst Excision

Clemente CD. Anatomy –a regional atlas of the human body. 4th ed. Baltimore: Williams and Wilkins; 1997.

Jamieson GG. The anatomy of general surgical operations. 2nd ed. Edinburgh: Churchill Livingston; 2006.

Submandibular Gland Excision

Clemente CD. Anatomy – a regional atlas of the human body. 4th ed. Baltimore: Williams and Wilkins; 1997.

Cunning DM, Lipke N, Wax MK. Significance of unilateral submandibular gland excision on salivary flow in noncancer patients. Laryngoscope. 1998;108(6):812–5.

Graham RM, Baldwin AJ. An unusual cause of Frey syndrome. Br J Oral Maxillofac Surg. 2009;47(2):146–7.

Jamieson GG. The anatomy of general surgical operations. 2nd ed. Edinburgh: Churchill Livingston; 2006.

Kowalski LP, Sanabria A. Elective neck dissection in oral carcinoma: a critical review of the evidence. Acta Otorhinolaryngol Ital. 2007;27(3):113–7.

Layfield LJ, Gopez E, Hirschowitz S. Cost efficiency analysis for fine-needle aspiration in the workup of parotid and submandibular gland nodules. Diagn Cytopathol. 2006;34(11):734–8.

Persaud NA, Myer 3rd CM, Rutter MJ. Gustatory sweating syndrome of the submandibular gland. Ear Nose Throat J. 2000;79(2):111–2.

Roh JL. Removal of the submandibular gland by a submental approach: a prospective, randomized, controlled study. Oral Oncol. 2008;44(3):295–300.

Roh JL, Choi SH, Lee SW, Cho KJ, Nam SY, Kim SY. Carcinomas arising in the submandibular gland: high propensity for systemic failure. J Surg Oncol. 2008;97(6):533–7.

Spiro RH. Salivary neoplasms: overview of a 35-year experience with 2,807 patients. Head Neck Surg. 1986;8(3):177–84.

Terhaard CH, Lubsen H, Rasch CR, Levendag PC, Kaanders HH, Tjho-Heslinga RE, van Den Ende PL, Burlage F, Dutch Head and Neck Oncology Cooperative Group. The role of radiotherapy in the treatment of malignant salivary gland tumors. Int J Radiat Oncol Biol Phys. 2005;61(1):103–11.

Torroni AA, Mustazza MC, Bartoli DD, Iannetti GG. Transcervical submandibular sialoadenectomy. J Craniofac Surg. 2007;18(3):613–21.

Submandibular Duct Dilatation

Clemente CD. Anatomy – a regional atlas of the human body. 4th ed. Baltimore: Williams and Wilkins; 1997.

Jamieson GG. The anatomy of general surgical operations. 2nd ed. Edinburgh: Churchill Livingston; 2006.

Branchial Cyst/Sinus Excision

Clemente CD. Anatomy – a regional atlas of the human body. 4th ed. Baltimore: Williams and Wilkins; 1997.

Jamieson GG. The anatomy of general surgical operations. 2nd ed. Edinburgh: Churchill Livingston; 2006.
Moore KL. The developing human – clinically oriented embryology. 2nd ed. Philadelphia: WB Saunders; 1977.

Mucous Cyst Excision of Lip/Cheek

Clemente CD. Anatomy – a regional atlas of the human body. 4th ed. Baltimore: Williams and Wilkins; 1997.
Jamieson GG. The anatomy of general surgical operations. 2nd ed. Edinburgh: Churchill Livingston; 2006.

Index

B.J. Coventry (ed.), *Peripheral, Head and Neck Surgery*,
Surgery: Complications, Risks and Consequences,
DOI 10.1007/978-1-4471-5415-0, © Springer-Verlag London 2014